Success in Academic Surgery

Series Editors

Lillian Kao
The University of Texas Health Science Centre
Houston, Texas
USA

Herbert Chen
Department of Surgery
University of Alabama at Birmingham
Birmingham, Alabama
USA

Melina R. Kibbe • Herbert Chen
Editors

Leadership in Surgery

Second Edition

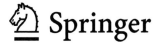 Springer

Editors
Melina R. Kibbe
Department of Surgery
University of North Carolina
Chapel Hill, NC
USA

Herbert Chen
Department of Surgery
University of Alabama at Birmingham
Birmingham, AL
USA

ISSN 2194-7481   ISSN 2194-749X   (electronic)
Success in Academic Surgery
ISBN 978-3-030-19853-4   ISBN 978-3-030-19854-1   (eBook)
https://doi.org/10.1007/978-3-030-19854-1

This Springer imprint is published by the registered company Springer Nature Switzerland AG
The registered company address is: Gewerbestrasse 11, 6330 Cham, Switzerland

Foreword

The visitor asked if any great men or women were born in this town. The reply was "No, only babies." While DNA may be important in determining some parts of human behavior and capabilities, life experiences and learning add crucial finishing touches. Leadership skills can be developed with conscious attention and understanding of the relevant principles and concepts. This book is a unique collection of pearls for surgeons from surgeons, the product of the experiences of current successful leaders, not just outside observers and behavioralists. Beyond a general discussion of what makes leadership and leaders, this second edition of a successful book explores the practical challenges faced in building teams, managing conflict, making the case for change, and navigating healthcare systems with a diverse surgical workforce. While directed at surgeons aspiring to rise in academic environments, it is applicable to surgical practices broadly.

American College of Surgeons   Andrew L. Warshaw
Chicago, IL, USA

Preface

The reason we decided to put this book together is because of a lack of leadership books and resources written by surgeons for surgeons. For this reason, we are very happy to offer the second edition of the *Leadership in Surgery* book. Leading in surgery does require not only common leadership skills but also subtle nuances and variations that do not apply consistently across all disciplines. These differences are expressed in the chapters of this book. In this second edition, many of the authors of the first edition have updated their chapters and continue to provide invaluable advice. We have included additional chapters on areas that any leader can benefit from in the present climate. We hope that you will find this book as valuable as we do.

Chapel Hill, NC   Melina R. Kibbe
Birmingham, AL   Herbert Chen

Contents

Barbara Lee Bass

What Is leadership?

Both a set of personal attributes and a collection of human behaviors, leadership is a complex combination of human qualities and actions. The primary purpose and value of a leader and leadership practice is to inspire others, deemed followers, to willingly engage together to achieve a goal. Leadership is a process and a trait which over the millennia of human society has assumed many forms in different cultures and organizations, from authoritative to democratic to communal. The valued human attributes of leaders and leadership, in the context of history, society, or organizations are inexorably shaped by time and place.

In this book we address leadership in the context of the contemporary academic healthcare department and system. This complex human performance enterprise whose primary mission is to provide healthcare to human beings, fortunately is motivated by a high moral purpose—healing—a mission which intrinsically inspires individuals to perform a service to others whatever their role in the organization. Further augmenting the missions of an academic healthcare system are the requirements to educate and train future generations of health care providers, in the case of surgery, future physicians and surgeons, as well as to expand the scientific knowledge and translational application of discovery to human health care. Serving these missions of intrinsic moral and human good would, hopefully, inspire effective and

B. L. Bass (⊠)
Department of Surgery, Houston Methodist Hospital, Houston, TX, USA

Houston Methodist Institute for Academic Medicine, Weill Cornell Medical College, Houston, TX, USA

Houston Methodist Institute for Technology, Innovation and Education (MITIE), Houston, TX, USA
e-mail: bbass@houstonmethodist.org

© Springer Nature Switzerland AG 2019
M. R. Kibbe, H. Chen (eds.), *Leadership in Surgery*, Success in Academic
Surgery, https://doi.org/10.1007/978-3-030-19854-1_1

value-based leaders. However, the challenges of leadership in modern healthcare systems are many with tough choices required by leaders regarding resource allocation, prioritization of mission, ongoing engagement of followers in personally demanding positions, and the increasing burden of emotional exhaustion fueled by advancement of technology and call for excessive human effort, all posing real threats to positive forward-looking leadership.

As with any complex human performance system, our academic healthcare environments are typically encumbered by layers of hierarchical structures, an infinite array of individuals with expertise across many disciplines—clinical, administrative, support industries, and others, factors that create challenges for organizations to form and execute high-performance teams in our health care ecosystems. Finding even shared language and core knowledge among the diverse populations that comprise the human workforce of an academic medical center is challenging. Nonetheless integrating the individual members of these component parts into effective, positive high-performance teams to deliver on the core mission of providing healthcare in an academic setting is essential to the success of the organizational mission. It is the job of leaders, built into the many layers of these systems, to guide the participants (and at times to be led as followers themselves) with whom they work into cohesive groups that willingly and indeed with great enthusiasm deliver on these missions.

Yet, this transformational time in healthcare, driven by the essential requirement to re-engineer delivery of healthcare around the needs of increasingly complex patients, rather than traditional physician driven models, requires fresh structures, units, processes and yes, high performance teams of non-traditional composition. It is the job of leadership to provide inspirational guidance and enabling motivation of the individuals who comprise the patient care delivery team, the educators, and the discoverers and translational investigators of our healthcare systems. Skilled and effective leaders will inspire and guide their followers, their diverse teams, to deliver on this mission of high moral value, despite these many challenges. This is the environment of leadership for those who rise or find themselves as leaders in modern healthcare institutions [1].

In this chapter we will examine the attributes of successful leaders in complex academic healthcare environments. What are the essential traits and qualities of leaders to serve as successful leaders? We will additionally explore the process of successful leadership. How does a leader motivate one's followers, one's team, to optimal performance? What are the steps and tools a leader may use to execute the job of leadership to motivate the modern health care team to serve the mission with enthusiasm, energy and excellence? We will explore these questions in this opening chapter.

The Attributes of Leaders

While leaders in many domains were once elevated into their roles as a heritable opportunity (or duty), in our modern healthcare system leaders now find themselves intentionally placed in positions of leadership by professional desire, ambition, and records of prior accomplishment. Leadership in our professional construct is allocated to or fallen upon an individual who has either by self-elevation, selection by his or her group, or by appointment by authorities of higher rank in an organization willingly agreed to take on the responsibility of serving as a leader.

We have long conventionally considered leadership in academic health care systems to be held by those with appointed roles of institutional authority—those with resource control opportunities and with decision making capacity related to policy, hiring, or strategy. As we will see however, surgeons and physicians in the culture of medicine are intrinsically recognized as leaders, both as primary holders and independent servants of their own patients' care but also as the final arbiters of clinical decision making among multi-disciplinary health care teams. We will explore the notion of leaders and leadership both as leaders in complex organizations, and physicians as leaders embedded in clinical environments in their daily workplaces. Both venues call for surgeons as leaders and the practice of leadership.

Interestingly, the qualities of leaders in professional, societal or governmental organizations were once aligned in gendered terms. Men were more likely to seek and to serve as leaders particularly in professional disciplines with historical longstanding gender imbalance of its members, such as academic surgery and other medical disciplines or more broadly in executive leadership in business and the legal profession, expectations for success and leadership were previously largely sought by and available to men. Concomitantly, the attributes of leaders once considered essential to success in these professions, including our own discipline—authoritative, decisive, self-confident, action oriented—have long been gendered attributes linked to male behaviors. To be a successful leader until recent years one had to take charge, direct, and inspire by sheer force of nature, power and personality. These were considered attributes of a successful leader which, certainly in hindsight, carried implicit male gendered linkage [2, 3].

However, these last two decades have seen a rethinking of the key attributes of successful leaders. Indeed, the gendered traits which in the past were linked to feminine qualities—collaborative, empathic, relational, enabling—have now been recognized as essential qualities of a successful leader in the academic healthcare industry and other professional environments. An effective and successful leader improves human performance by inspiring others to work together, leveraging the talents of a diverse workforce, to create the working unit of healthcare delivery. Today's successful academic healthcare leaders, men and women, exhibit the traits once collectively linked to feminine attributes that are distinctly related to forming meaningful connections between people, between themselves as leaders and those who they are charged to lead. Qualities of leadership that foster inclusion and engagement are now prioritized as values and are embraced as non-gendered behaviors.

In addition to these human connection qualities to enable effective leaders, core successful attributes of leaders today include integrity, authenticity, honesty, and fairness. These attributes must intrinsically be accompanied by a leader's competence in their position and a commitment to the collective effort of the organization. Coupling these attributes to qualities of positive energy, forward-looking optimism and resilience lead to a clear structure of an inspiring leader.

A most powerful pool of leadership is humility. Humility is that trait which allows a leader to recognize his or her own limitations, to acknowledge error, and to respect the wisdom of others. Collectively these very human qualities and attributes are consistent with our shared moral framework of positive human attributes. A good leader is admired for his or her abilities and attributes and when coupled to execution of leadership to deliver a compelling vision and desirable mission, fosters engagement of the followers in the team. Collectively these human attributes when utilized for the good of the organization inspire followers who will willingly and energetically work together as teams to deliver on mission.

Bundled into an operational construct, these attributes of human connectivity are often described in the framework of emotional intelligence. More extensively considered in a later chapter, emotional intelligence is that personal attribute that enables human: human interaction in social and professional environments. The fundamental elements of emotional intelligence include a practice of recognizing one's own response to situational events, a phenomenon known as self-awareness. Individuals with abundant emotional intelligence are aware of their own emotional reactions to life events particularly as they relate to their interactions with other people. Emotional intelligence also encompasses the ability to be self aware of how one's speech and performance and interaction may impact others; the ability to recognize the impact of a human social exchange on oneself and to observe and understand the impact on the other party. Critical to high-performing emotional intelligence is the ability to understand the thoughts and feelings of others and to recognize with empathy the impact of events or interactions on others [4].

Being able to understand others' feelings and perspectives in a supportive and empathic way enables human connection and is key to success as a leader in our modern healthcare academic setting, an environment that relies on collective efforts of teams of individuals to optimize the delivery of quality patient care. All of us can recall the brilliant and capable individuals who failed as leaders not due to technical incompetence, but for their failure to engage the support and participation of their followers given their inability to understand human feelings and make meaningful connections. Having the skills of self-awareness, empathy, and self-regulation enable one as a leader to exert positive influence on others in a motivating and fair fashion. One aspires as a leader to elicit responsiveness and engagement in one's team or followers by understanding their motivation values and goals. Armed with these contextual emotional clues a leader can motivate optimal human performance by others.

The Practice of Leadership

Leadership is an active process. Spanning many domains of action, the most fundamental responsibilities of leadership are to articulate the vision to serve the purpose of the organization the leader serves. Coupled with equal responsibility to this vision setting is to delineate the missions of the organization to achieve that visionary goal. In our academic healthcare environments, this vision and mission, is fundamentally fortunately linked as we have noted previously, to a valuable societal good, providing care to the sick, injured and frail among us. We are additionally charged with raising the healthcare and surgical workforce of the future who will carry this mission in the decades ahead, another shared societal value. And we are charged with discovery of new knowledge to benefit human health and develop new modalities and interventions to improve the care we provide, thus completing the threesome of societal benefits our organizations are charged to deliver. These are certainly uniformly agreeable morally high purpose missions [5].

Yet today's healthcare leaders are also required to articulate and deliver on this mission in the modern context of resource limitations, equity of access, patient primacy, and intentional inclusion of diverse populations and voices. We work in an environment of scalable complexity from the very personal one on one patient physician encounter to the multibillion-dollar healthcare systems where we practice our art and leadership in interchanges that reflect not individual moments, but population driven exchanges. Maintaining moral purpose at interfaces that are more remote from individual human acts can be challenging, less obviously humanizing, but is an essential skilled practice of good leaders.

The effective practice of leadership is informed by the limitations of the resources and environment of the organization in which the followers, the team members, will work. While in extraordinary or threatening times, directive and authoritarian leadership styles may be required; in less stressed moments, effective leadership knows to set mission goals, both short and long-term, that may be achieved with available resources and within the talents of the organization team members. Stretch goals are often positive motivators for teams, but good leadership recognizes that relentless expectations for success in environments where resources and structures are oppressive, will elicit frustration and ineffective engagement of the team of followers [5].

Leadership is a process of engagement. Effective leadership elicits willingness, indeed eagerness, to those within the group to work together to achieve the mission. Good leadership articulates the positive value of the contributions of the members of the team. While many incentives may facilitate engagement of the members to work collectively and individually to achieve the goals and certainly equitable and fair compensation is essential, exclusive financial drivers, avoidance of negative consequences, and token personal promotions are rarely sustainable sufficient motivators in high-performance organizations. The most effective leadership creates a shared sense of purpose and value, a motivating reward is more that transactional acknowledgement of hitting a target. Rather the reward is a shared sense of accomplishment—a we did it moment—on having completed a mission driven my positive shared purpose, a "good" purpose. No more clear an example of the motivating value of shared vision and purpose, not financial reward or personal recognition, to deliver on mission can be identified than the collective energy and contributions of those individuals who worked at NASA during the years of the lunar exploration flights.

The notion of value-based leadership, to achieve a laudable good, may be confounding. In the business world, shared values may be reflected in financial terms, market share, visibility. In the healthcare sector of academic surgery and medicine, value-based leadership requires greater clarity on the notion of "good". Leadership in academic departments of surgery must additionally motivate the missions of education and discovery. In today's health care systems with financial engines acutely tuned to the clinical delivery of care, these important additional missions may face genuine challenges. The value of good stewardship is fundamental to leadership in academic surgical environments. Financial security, minimization of waste and redundancy, efficiency, all factors which lead to a positive financial value, are aspects of organizational performance that are often viewed as irritants in a team's work. Leaders must articulate to persuade one's teams that these processes and goals are indeed core elements of good stewardship and leadership in academic departments, processes that assure that these other essential missions can be augmented and supported.

Leadership is service to others. Yes, most certainly, leaders are the recipients of substantial benefits by the authority and responsibility vested in them by their organizational roles. The rewards include financial benefit, access to privileged organizational information, recognition in the community and one's profession, and hopefully respect for one's performance as a leader. Leaders' voices are heard and acknowledged, at times justifiably by content and wise contributions, but at times simply by position. These are the rewards and respect that are given to leaders during their tenures. One hopes that these rewards are justifiable, well-earned, and of intrinsic reward to the leader.

But fundamentally, modern leadership that is effective and rightfully privileged, is not based on authority of position but rather on the practice of leadership demonstrating commitment and the energetic ability to serve the mission and purpose of the organization and to facilitate the service provided by the assembled teams to achieve goals. The role of a leader, at its core, is to serve the needs of others.

Leadership and Teams

The current construct of an ideal operational group in healthcare is a multidisciplinary team. The team has members with distinct functional responsibilities and talent and diversity of perspective and abilities. High-performing teams synergistically bring individual strengths and talents to execute the actions of the group to achieve the mission. Good leaders of teams, in fact, enhance the strengths of teams and improve the individual member's sense of worth and purpose by allowing various members to intrinsically "take the lead". Mutual respect for the skills, talents, and perspectives of the team members is essential to high team performance. Rotating leadership, recognizing distinct expertise within a team may not only build trust among the team members, but also improve the delivery goals.

Modern healthcare, particularly in the setting of academic healthcare systems requires many types of expertise to deliver on mission. Physicians and surgeons, nurses, pharmacists, technologists, social support professionals, administrative support staff, executive staff members—each brings expertise and expectations for contributions to the delivery of quality patient care. Nonetheless, the power of the physician voice as a leader carries special weight in most healthcare environments.

Wittingly, or otherwise, physicians bear a special responsibility in creating the new environment of leadership needed in the academic health care setting. There is a shared collective notion in most complex health care settings of final authority for physicians in matters of clinical decision making and creation of treatment pathways. While not clearly codified at times, this venue is likely the most common form of leadership that surgeons and physicians encounter in their professional roles: the assumed and valued leader in the clinical microcosm of the health care delivery team.

Yet, we have not taught surgeons and physicians how to engage as leaders in these multidisciplinary teams. Physicians and surgeons are raised as highly autonomous practitioners: the surgeon is solely responsible for her or his patient. While recent medical and graduate medical education curricula have introduced constructs to improve the performance of surgeons as effective team members (yes, at times to be followers) and as leaders, the longstanding practice of physician primacy fueled by that pathway of individual accomplishment and drive, has been hard to overcome and rarely incorporated into daily training practices [6, 7].

Best practices for clinician leaders in clinical microcosm teams have been articulated. Given their inherent opportunity for recognition as a leader in the clinical microcosm, physicians and surgeons have an exceptional ability to impact care processes and strategies in a multidisciplinary team. Though often without designated title or explicit resource control, physician leaders in these distinctly mission focused teams can provide the guiding vision and value for achieving important patient care goals at the organizational level. The lack of physician participation and indeed leadership dooms most clinical change or improvement efforts to the margins of engagement and likely failure. Physicians and surgeon leaders can demonstrate and hold significant power in implementing important changes in the microcosm, simply by demonstrating genuine engaged behaviors—endorsement of the value of the mission, expression of genuine curiosity about best strategy and process to engage the team to achieve what may be a formidable improvement, recognition of the challenges faced to achieve goal and time burden placed on those in the microcosm to deliver on goal. Effective leadership in these clinical microcosms is a new model of leadership for surgeons in academic environments which call for humility, respect and belief in the talents of others, and relentless positive energy to promote collective action which almost certainly calls for ceding of leadership roles to others on the team at various steps along the way. Surgeon leadership practiced at the highest level in this manner allows all members of the team to participate in the joy of achieving a goal and to have contributed in so doing, inspired energy and future engagement for all [8–10].

Leadership is informed by humility. In high-performance, complex human activity environments, error in judgment and execution by a leader are inevitable. No vision is perfect, even in hindsight. A good leader is aware and willing to acknowledge his or her personal error in judgment or performance, to apologize as needed, to seek counsel to repair damage and to restore a positive course to allow the organization to move forward with new energy and direction. A trusted leader will be given these opportunities to fail and then to recover. A leader who has led lacking integrity or with self-serving intent, will not be allowed the opportunity to recover.

Challenges to Leadership

Leading in Times of Crisis

Leadership during times of crisis, of which there are many forms, is particularly challenging. Times of crisis elicit uncertainty, fear, and anxiety in individuals and collectively in the organization. These human reactions to crisis intrinsically affect not only the organization but also the leader personally. It is during these periods when perhaps the genuine attributes of leaders are most clear. Certainly, the need for effective leadership is indeed clear at times of crisis.

Crises can take many forms. Personal loss, including loss of valued members of the organization or team to injury, illness, or even suicide, the most devastating and challenging loss for an organization to sustain. Organizational instability, a change in leadership or restructuring, or financial instability can create a sense of crisis and panic in an organization and its members. Natural disasters or national crises of horrific events can each bring potential instability and insecurity to an organization or an organization's workforce. It is during these hard times that leaders must exhibit and practice their skills of leadership most profoundly.

Tools of leadership during times of crises require an investment of greater personal energy. While the leader to may be feeling the insecurity and anxiety and fear of the event at hand, a leader, unless truly disabled oneself, will be able to call upon the tools of personal values to guide the organization through the crisis. Times of crisis calls for more open expression of empathy, humility, and expression of concerns. However, the job of leadership is also to put forward the face of resilience and forward thinking optimism and problem solving in times of crisis. It is a time when leaders even more actively engage the collective strength and wisdom of their teams to enable the organization to move into recovery or repair mode. It is a time when hierarchy is flattened as one deals with more forward facing human concerns. Leadership may be most challenging during these times, but once the crisis ebbs and recovery begins, the rewards of engaging collective wisdom and energy become clear and most gratifying.

Breaches of Professionalism

Old constructs of authoritative leadership, surgeons as the timeless captains of the ship, present real challenges to effective leadership in the modern healthcare system. While it is true that no patient comes to the operating room to receive an anesthetic procedure, the surgery that that patient did submit to cannot be accomplished without the benefit of the anesthetic team. Surgeons once balked at requirements for timeouts, metrics of antibiotic administration, antithrombotic guideline use, noting that in their own experience that their patients did not suffer adverse outcomes of wrong site surgery, preventable wound infections or deep vein thrombosis. The abundant evidence of best practice however, has now revealed the value to these practices as applied in a high-performance system of surgical care—a team-based event.

The surgeon who harshly admonishes operating room staff or anesthesia colleagues in the interest of protecting their patient, creating tension and fearfulness in the team, in fact creates an environment that fosters flawed performance by all.

Surgical leaders have the particular mission to ensure professionalism in the complex team based environments of the medical center: the operating rooms, emergency department, SICU and other areas. This task is often complicated once again by the surgeon primacy culture—allowing that aggressive surgeon behavior was fueled not by anger but by the surgeon's passion for caring for his or her patient when all others seems to have abandoned that responsibility. Clearly, such abandonment is exceedingly rare among our skilled colleagues of other disciplines. It is the job of institutional surgical leadership to repair the disruptive and broken behaviors in these dysfunctional teams in surgical environments. The institution leadership is faced with the challenge of engaging surgeons, long accustomed to primacy, to function in more horizontal teams and indeed to adopt new patterns of respect for the other professionals in the health care team. Simulation based training has been a recent tool to foster this enhanced teamwork.

As a first step, surgical leaders must lead by example in the domain of professionalism. Intolerance of harassing, predatory or unprofessional behaviors in the surgical healthcare environment cannot be condoned in any form. One of the harder jobs of leadership is to ensure that such behaviors are excluded in our patient care and educational environments, for such behaviors not only create victims, but also diminish the ability of professional teams to practice at a high-quality level. Disruptive physicians disrupt everyone and everything.

Leading Up

Everyone in an organization has a boss. The CEO and president have the Board, the Dean the President, the Executive vice president the CEO, the chairs and center directors—all of the above! Successful leaders at each level recognize that to optimize their performance as leaders of the groups and tasks they are assigned to guide, their vision and mission must be reasonably concordant with those of the organization from the top down. For chairs as leaders, the task is dually complex. As positioned in the organization, chairs have not only leadership functions at the highly personal level of patient care, faculty selection and development, resident and medical surgent engagement, and often as a researcher, but also as an institutional steward of valuable resources and executors of organizational goals; i.e. personal engagement skills and executive leadership skills are both vitally important. Leading up requires not only awareness and engagement in delivering the institutional missions, but also awareness of the leadership styles and qualities of those to whom one reports. Creating an environment that enables trust and ongoing investment from the leaders to whom one reports relies on a leader's core competence to deliver on mission, engagement and positive performance of the many teams one has crafted and set on mission, and demonstration of success as a respected and trusted leader of those one is charged to guide as a leader. Effective leaders in organizations, from the surgeons in the clinical microcosm, to the chair of the department or executive vice president or dean, regardless of their hierarchical position, launch forward looking initiatives, engage in creative solution solving to serve the organizational needs and goals, and work within the framework of the organization's leadership to collectively move the institution forward.

Summary

In summary, leadership is both a daunting and gratifying process. Good leadership serves a shared moral purpose to serve laudable goals in concert with engaged followers. In the academic health care system, good leadership will provide a positive, forward looking vision to optimize delivery of the missions of quality patient care, education and discovery and create an environment of empowerment for the multidisciplinary teams who are the fabric of the academic health system. To be successful, leaders must inspire the complex human performance teams in our health care systems—including those tasked with the least empowered roles to the most privileged participants—to work collectively to deliver those missions. Great leaders inspire by qualities of personal integrity, competence, honesty, and human connection with and service to those they lead and the mission they serve. Leaders will face difficult decisions regarding priority setting, and during times of change or crisis, but adherence to a moral compass coupled to shared values, respect for others, and humility will allow a leader to create a pathway of optimism that will inspire others to work positively and optimally together to achieve shared goals.

References

1. Goleman D. What makes a leader? Harv Bus Rev. 1 Jan 2004. p. 1–12.
2. Zenger J, Folkman J. Are women better leaders than men. Harv Bus Rev. 15 Mar 2012.
3. Gerzema DJ. The Athena Doctrine: how women (and the men who think like them) will rule the future. San Francisco: Jossey-Bass; 2013.
4. Goleman D, Boyatzis R, McKee A. Primal leadership: realizing the power of emotional intelligence. Boston: Harvard Business Press; 2002.
5. Goleman D. Leadership that gets results. Harv Bus Rev. 1 Apr 2000.
6. Bohmer RMJ. Leading clinicians and clinicians leading. N Engl J Med. 2013;368(16):1468–70.
7. Eddy K, Jordan Z, Stephenson M. Health professionals' experience of teamwork education in acute hospital settings: a systematic review of qualitative literature. JBI Database System Rev Implement Rep. 2016;14:96–137.
8. Sadowski B, Cantrell S, Barelski A, O'Malley PG, Hartzell JD. Leadership training in graduate medical education: a systematic review. J Grad Med Educ. 2018;10:134–48.
9. Steinert Y, Naismith L, Mann K. Faculty development initiatives designed to promote leadership in medical education. Med Teach. 2012;34:483–503.
10. Lee TH. Turning doctors into leaders. Harv Bus Rev. 2010;88:50–8.

Michael Mulholland

Surgical Leadership in a Time of Change

Surgery currently holds a central place in the complex American health care system, but change is everywhere. Approximately 100 million procedures are performed annually by 275,000 surgical specialists. Surgical services are expensive, costing $500 billion each year, and operative procedures are uniquely remunerative to hospitals, typically accounting for 40% of hospital revenue. The technical aspects of surgical practice have evolved very rapidly in the two decades since the widespread adoption of laparoscopic cholecystectomy. Laparoscopic approaches have supplanted most open operations, now joined by thoracoscopy, endovascular therapy, and image-guided surgery. Scientific advances have also changed the intellectual underpinnings of surgical practice. Insights into the structure and function of the human genome are reflected in personalized medicine, to be joined shortly by personalized surgical therapy. Postgraduate surgical training has been forced to evolve as techniques and knowledge have changed, creating both opportunities and new challenges. The surgical workforce has changed tremendously over the past 10–15 years, both demographically and in practice phenotype.

Effective surgical leadership is required for Surgery to remain relevant to the future practice of medicine. Failing that, Surgery may be reduced to a technical specialty, and vulnerable to loss of identity and to displacement from decision making regarding delivery of care. Surgical leadership must be future-oriented, applying lessons from the past to circumstances yet to come. At its best, leadership involves creation of a positive future by communicating the idea that cooperative, team-based behavior always achieves more than individual or self-motivated behavior. Leaders create the future by:

M. Mulholland (✉)
Department of Surgery, University of Michigan, Ann Arbor, MI, USA
e-mail: micham@med.umich.edu

© Springer Nature Switzerland AG 2019
M. R. Kibbe, H. Chen (eds.), *Leadership in Surgery*, Success in Academic Surgery, https://doi.org/10.1007/978-3-030-19854-1_2

1. Developing a compelling vision;
2. Communicating a positive view of future possibilities;
3. Seeking consensus in support of that vision;
4. Developing diverse talent needed for the pursuit of future accomplishments;
5. Demonstrating commitment over time to achievement of that vision.

The Leadership Imperative

As a first step in considering surgical leadership, it is important to consider the activities with which surgeons are engaged, and then to ask how these tasks promote leadership.

The Clinical Mission

Surgeons express the clinical mission in care of individual patients and health systems are organized to facilitate the provision of operative care. Operating room suites are central physical features of every hospital in this country. Operating room construction is highly regulated and uniquely expensive, making disproportionate claims on hospital capital and operating funds. Personnel requirements exceed those of other areas of hospital operations, magnified by the 24/7 nature of surgical activity at most large hospitals. In addition, operating room functions make large demands upon other services, including radiology, blood banking, and pathology. In many systems, ambulatory clinics and emergency rooms are explicitly designed to efficiently funnel patients to surgical providers.

Within this system, surgeons have possessed unique degrees of professional autonomy and flexibility. Anesthesiologists, operating room nurses and surgical support personnel are assigned to a daily surgical schedule and are committed to finishing the cases presented. With many fewer constraints, surgeons may schedule elective operations at their discretion and in ways that maximize professional gain while minimizing personal conflicts. Surgeons are allowed greater degrees of freedom in equipment and supply requests than other physicians. For example, most operating rooms maintain an extensive list of "doctor preference cards" that outline the needs of each surgeon for commonly performed operations, the preferences often substantially different for operations that are largely similar. Even though operating room personnel are highly skilled and expensive, surgery does not begin until the surgeon is ready. As these few examples illustrate, the operating room is a highly artificial environment designed to maximize productivity of surgeons. Unfortunately, these hierarchical aspects of surgical care, long part of surgical culture, are not conducive to leadership development. This autocratic form of surgical leadership, so common in the past, is rapidly vanishing and is being replaced instead by a collaborative culture based on open communication and mutual respect.

Within the operating room, the importance of communication and interpersonal relationships has been recognized in recent years through team-building efforts.

Surgical checklists, pre-incision time outs and postoperative debriefing are all expressions of the same incredibly simple, but powerful idea: every member of a surgical team has unique insights and value is gained by sharing information. The results have been impressive. As reported by the Safe Surgery Saves Lives Study Group, the institution of a multidisciplinary surgical safety checklist, including medications, marking of the operative site and postoperative instructions significantly improved operative results [1].

Surgical care is now multidisciplinary care. Long the domain of surgical oncologists and transplant surgeons, multidisciplinary clinics and case conferences increasingly dominate cardiovascular surgery, bariatric surgery, pediatric surgery, and many other disciplines. Success in multidisciplinary settings requires the practitioner to be knowledgeable of the others' disciplines, to appreciate and respect alternative perspectives, to resolve clinical ambiguity and to engage in multilateral negotiation. These attributes are precisely the characteristics required for modern surgical leadership.

Surgical leaders must interpret the demands of surgery to others. Provision of surgical care is resource and capital intensive and may conflict with other health system demands. For example, in hospitals with high occupancy, admissions from the emergency department may compete for beds devoted to elective surgical cases. Ongoing changes in hospital reimbursement shift financial risk progressively to health systems and may convert surgical services from revenue generating units to cost centers. Adoption of bundled payment systems will require substantial internal readjustments. The interpersonal skills exemplified by multidisciplinary care are directly relevant to navigating these coming changes.

Most importantly, surgical leaders must imagine and empower a future in which treatment of the next generation of patients is better than contemporary care.

The Research Mission

In academic medical centers, innovation is the chief source of differentiation and competitive advantage, and surgeons must actively engage in scientific discovery to remain relevant. In contemporary basic investigation, however, there is no surgical research, just research. Basic investigation is reductionist and mechanistically oriented. Western blotting and polymerase chain reaction and transgenic animal models apply equally to investigators from Surgery, Immunology or Biochemistry. In addition, methodological advances in genetics, metabolomics and biocomputation, among many others, make it impossible for any single investigator to master all techniques. Basic science is now and forever a team sport. As such, success in basic science requires equal measures of analytic talent and personality. As clinical medicine has become multidisciplinary, so too has biology.

Similar changes have occurred in clinical and health services research. The performance of an operation constitutes a clear transition in care, and a cause and effect relationship between intervention and outcomes like complication or death is less equivocal than for non-surgical treatment. The link between operation and outcome has been the intellectual lynchpin of surgical health services research. To date, the clarity of this relationship has allowed health services research to remain largely "surgical". This situation will not persist. The creation of national data repositories and the influence of ideas from economics and social research have changed and enriched this field. Soon there will be no surgical health services research, just health services research.

A uniquely powerful opportunity for surgical investigators exists at the intersection of health services research and quality improvement. The potential for large-scale collaborative investigation is exemplified by the Michigan Surgical Quality Collaborative (MSQC), a consortium of 72 hospitals in the state of Michigan, each led by a surgical champion (Fig. 2.1). The range of investigations undertaken by MSQC has spanned topics as varied as surgical infections, intraoperative technical coaching and economic analysis. The MSQC has also spawned other large-scale, high-impact research collaboratives with direct relevance to contemporary patient care, for example the Michigan Opioid Prescribing Engagement Network (M-OPEN). The motto of these groups is compelling: Collaboration is the New Competition.

An inevitable tension exists between the clear demands and tangible rewards of clinical surgery and the uncertainty of research. A long line of past patients and a seemingly unlimited number of future patients confront the surgeon. The emergency department demands attention every day. The emotional rewards of a well-executed operation are immediate. Financial results are obvious. In contrast, novel ideas are fleeting and rare. Surgical leaders can shape the research mission through personal research accomplishments and scholarship. They also support investigation by displaying intellectual engagement, perseverance and curiosity. As with clinical care, surgical leaders must imagine and fund future investigation.

Fig. 2.1 Patient care collaboratives in Michigan

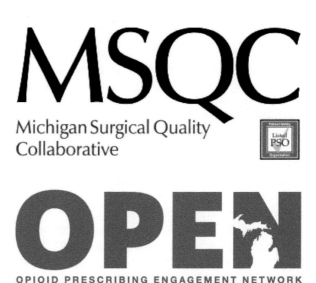

The Teaching Mission

Surgeons involved in undergraduate medical education and in postgraduate training are uniquely privileged. Beyond the patients they treat directly, these individuals influence the lives of thousands of others, cared for in turn by their trainees. Cognitive development in surgical training is not different from that associated with other medical disciplines. The principles of adult learning apply equally to both groups of learners. In contrast, the technical aspects of surgical training have no parallels in non-surgical disciplines. The teaching of surgery requires special traits of the instructor—patience, the ability to instill confidence in another person, communication through both verbal and non-verbal cues, and the self-possession required to help another succeed.

Training to be a surgeon can be emotionally trying, and not for the obvious reasons that the hours can be long and physically fatiguing or that surgical emergencies are stressful. Surgery is difficult because committing to an operation imparts responsibility to the surgeon for another person's life. Not all patients can be cured; palliation may be elusive; complications occur. Failure is intrinsic to the practice of surgery. The best teachers of surgery are empathic to their trainees and are able to guide emotional maturation. These traits are surely the substrate of leadership.

The Talent Development Mission

Surgical leaders are talent scouts. Most physicians are ultimately drawn to the intellectual foundations of the disciplines they choose, but many are initially attracted to the field by the example of a more senior mentor. Talented young people are stimulated by environments that are open, accepting of differences and rewarding. A small research project becomes a presentation at a symposium, which begets a larger project, which blossoms into an investigative career.

For any department of surgery, success is due to the talent, commitment, and vision of its faculty. A crucial role of surgical leadership is to help every individual develop to his or her full potential. The mission should be to:

1. Prepare each surgeon to achieve the highest excellence in clinical care, research, and education.
2. Build a diverse and inclusive culture in which all individuals advance and thrive.
3. Recruit the best and brightest clinicians and scientists.
4. Create innovative strategies for ongoing professional growth and scientific discovery.
5. Mentor and sponsor diverse phenotypes to enhance cognitive diversity and productivity.
6. Develop the most talented and progressive future leaders.
7. Expand outreach and service to local, regional, national, and global partners.

Fig. 2.2 The Michigan
Promise

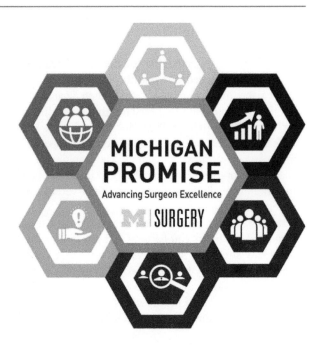

The Michigan Promise represents a longitudinal investment in the faculty of the Department of Surgery at the University of Michigan (Fig. 2.2). This multifaceted approach is designed to encompass these missions. The Michigan Promise is a long-term commitment to faculty development and an effort to change the face of American Surgery for the next generation. There are six areas of focus—Environment, Achievement, Leadership, Recruitment, Innovation and Outreach.

For these missions, defined strategies exist within these domains with each initiative open to all faculty members within the department across rank, track, and specialty. The Michigan Promise is designed to accelerate achievement and ensure that the environment allows all individuals to achieve excellence and professional satisfaction. Because faculty play a central role in executing the mission of the Department of Surgery, these efforts are integrated as a core value of equal importance to other core departmental values. Each initiative within the Michigan Promise is coordinated and executed through the Department of Surgery Office of Faculty Life, addressing challenges of achieving excellence in clinical care, teaching, research, diversity, and equity in modern academic medicine.

Diversity, equity and inclusion are an explicit part of The Michigan Promise. The faculty collectively believe in the power diversity—that combining different perspectives and integrating diverse cognitive repertoires is key to our future success. As one example to achieve this, the department created a committee tasked with overseeing all faculty recruitment. Members are trained in implicit bias awareness and are chosen to represent the diversity in the department. Candidate pools are enriched for diversity by outreach and interview processes and questions are standardized.

The program reinforces an open and welcoming environment in which everyone is provided the opportunity to advance and lead. To achieve this, the department has implemented implicit bias training and has been engaged heavily in consciousness raising. Leaders must ensure that individual barriers are addressed and eliminated, and that all individuals are empowered to reach their highest potential.

Leadership must ensure the intentional development of young faculty. To achieve this, the department provides launch teams; an early career Leadership Development Program; and an early career visiting professor program with partner institutions. Equally important is leadership development of mid-career and senior faculty. To achieve this, the department provides a unique Leadership Development Program; an Innovation Development Program with an Innovation Prize; an opportunity for a directed 2-month sabbatical to develop new skills; and Leadership Masters Classes.

These professional development programs are responsive to each faculty member's needs, and include support, mentorship, and sponsorship throughout an academic career. The programs are dynamic, and incorporate innovative strategies from other disciplines tailored to the demands of academic surgery. Through these efforts, the faculty should be well equipped and positioned to become leaders locally, nationally, and internationally.

Initial Faculty Experiences

During junior faculty years, those immediately following the completion of residency or fellowship training, formal administrative responsibilities should be minimized. Every surgeon upon entering independent practice must develop personal clinical judgment, determine how he will comport himself in an operating room, and must establish ties to referring physicians. Complications occur in every practice and the young surgeon must learn to face them forthrightly and with equanimity. In teaching hospitals, the young faculty member must switch from receiving instruction to providing guidance. The first years are especially important in research; lack of focus and productivity at this juncture can permanently short circuit an investigative career. In the most positive sense, these years should be a self-directed investment in future productivity. While many of these activities are the building blocks of leadership, and while every year provides opportunities for leadership, personal development requires time and focus.

Surgery is the most public form of medical practice. As an obvious example, surgical procedures are performed in an operating room with a scrub nurse and a circulating nurse, anesthesiology care giver and often one or more trainees. At another level, the direct relationship of surgical complications to the performance of an operation makes public examination of imperfect results routine. A weekly morbidity and mortality conference is a staple of every surgical training program in this country. The risk inherent to surgery, its public nature and the resultant scrutiny thrusts surgical leaders into positions of judgment. Credibility in this regard is contingent upon the leader's clinical abilities. Strong cultural norms in American Surgery make it very difficult for surgeons that are not clinically experienced and active to assume meaningful leadership roles.

Research is the key to improving current surgical practice. Investigation is also uncertain and expensive. Surgical research is not relevant to non-academic medical centers, and has become optional or endangered at many others. Where research is important, early investigative success is an essential criterion for surgical leadership.

Clinical teaching is less embattled than research and is a foundation of most departments of surgery. A commitment to teaching and a record of teaching ability should be considered a prerequisite to leadership development.

Temperament and Values

While experience is influential in leadership development, in many ways temperament is more important. To succeed in these dimensions, surgical leaders must possess integrity, humility, selflessness, the ability to communicate and curiosity.

Personal integrity is the single most important quality of leadership. While integrity alone does not guarantee leadership success, the perceived absence of this quality does guarantee failure. At the simplest level, integrity means that the effective leader does what he has said he will do. For example, if the surgical leader has committed to provide resources to a newly recruited faculty member, integrity means that those resources have been accrued and will be available. If a salary has been negotiated, the money will be paid. Operating room time promised will be delivered. Promises that are made for material or financial benefits will be met. However, integrity in this sense is purely transactional. Transactional interactions do not engage group imagination or collective action, and leadership that rests solely on the authority to provide material benefit or financial transfers is fragile [2].

Beyond transactional commitments, integrity means the group perceives that the leader does what she thinks is right. This state implies that the organization understands that the leader has a moral framework that informs decisions, is consistently true to those convictions, and that she resists powerful forces within the organization that threaten group welfare. Consider the promises alluded to above. In any surgical department, there is never enough lab space, money or operating room time to satisfy the needs and aspirations of all. Necessarily, commitment of resources to one faculty recruit, salary increase to another or operating room time to a third, affects the whole organization. In addition, there are no guarantees at the time of commitment that those resources will be used productively or to the benefit of the whole organization. Decisions of the leader that are seen to arise from a moral center of gravity allow the group to accept the risks that commitment of resources always entails.

At the highest level, personal integrity requires the explicit acknowledgement on the part of the leader that he or she is fallible. No single person can be fully informed on all subjects nor error-free. This perspective requires the leader to seek a broad range of views and to make important decisions only after considering multiple viewpoints. Public vulnerability by leaders is a powerful force within an organization. Vulnerability enables a fuller expression of ideas by all group members, especially junior faculty. The differing perspectives that emerge increase organizational performance and lead to improved efficiency, innovation and financial outcomes. This effect has been called cognitive diversity [3]. The power of cognitive diversity is grounded in leadership humility.

Integrity also has a time element. Personal integrity displayed over time creates trust. Trust is hard-earned, resilient, and very powerful in that this condition allows the group to engage with the leader's longer term vision. With trust, a belief develops that the leader will be consistent through success and failure, that the leader encountered today will express the same values in the future. Let the reader imagine a personal example. Think of a person in your life whom you trust. Imagine that you have not seen him or her in a month, a year, perhaps a decade. Trust means you believe that when you meet this person next he or she will display a consistent set of values and will treat you fairly, as you have been treated in the past.

Effective leaders work to achieve a vision for the future that maximizes the potential of others and benefits the organization, for example a department of surgery. To do so, the leader must be outward-looking and not concerned with personal advantage or benefit. There must be joy and satisfaction for the leader in the success and recognition of others. This quality of selflessness is a core ethical value in medicine in which the welfare and benefit of the patient takes precedence over the self-interest of the treating physician. This viewpoint is diametrically opposed to modern American business practices in which maximizing profit is the standard and in which placing personal interest first is an accepted ethical starting point. Selflessness cannot be taught. For surgical leaders, this quality requires a bedrock sense of personal wholeness and confidence.

Communication

Communication is absolutely essential to leadership. Effective leadership requires a commitment to continuous expression of core values, institutional objectives and future aspirations.

The most powerful communication resides in the manner in which a leader lives his or her life. For better and worse, leaders are observed and their actions (and inactions) are scrutinized. Respectful language, humility, and humane treatment of others' failings resonate strongly and positively. Positive communication of this sort allows the leader to accumulate credit in a bank of goodwill. This credit can be depleted incredibly rapidly, sometimes instantly, by crude humor, hubris, or cruelty. Perceived hypocrisy in a leader is especially corrosive. A leader cannot profess value in teaching and at the same time ignore medical students, and cannot ask others to be productive in research while not being academically engaged. The surgical leader's professional life is on brightest display in the operating room. The surgeon leader does not need to be the most technically gifted operator in the department, but he or she absolutely must be the most respectful to the nurses, the calmest when problems arise, the person with whom the anesthesiologists feel most comfortable. True surgical leadership cannot be gained solely in the operating room, but it can surely be lost.

In our verbal society, spoken communication is key, and effective leaders develop multiple styles of verbal expression. It seems obvious that talking privately with a junior house officer struggling with a major postoperative complication would differ in approach than annual salary negotiations with senior faculty. Public presentations to scientifically sophisticated professional audiences require different language skills than do talks to lay groups.

Effective communication uses a variety of verbal tools, and leaders must work to master all. Consider the power of analogy. This author might describe his work at a research seminar by saying "My laboratory studies hypothalamic control of ingestive behavior and metabolic rate. We have deep expertise in the melanocortin signaling system and have developed a number of transgenic animal models to examine signal transduction in this system." This description probably would not work with a successful business person considering laboratory endowment. Perhaps it might be better to say "I study eating. The brain has an area that acts like a thermostat. Turn the thermostat up and we feel hungry; turn it down and we stop eating. I'm trying to see if we can control that thermostat so we can cure overweight."

While verbal expression is important, listening is more important. Effective listening is not passive, and active listening is a skill that must be developed. Listening effectively involves asking questions as the other speaks to elicit deeper meaning, to clarify ambiguity and to draw forth new ideas. Active listening involves verbal encouragement and visual cues, and sometimes just sitting silently while the speaker organizes his or her thoughts. The best leaders practice a 2:1 rule; the leader listens 2 min for every minute that he or she talks. Listening is not easy; it requires practice.

Because we live in such a verbal/visual society, there is special power for leaders who can also express themselves in writing with style and clarity. Writing is hard work. Ann Patchett, the highly successful novelist, has recently written "Logic dictates that writing should be a natural act, a function of a well-operating human body, along the lines of speaking and walking and breathing. We should be able to tap into the constant narrative flow our minds provide, the roaring river of words filling up our heads, and direct it out into a neat stream of organized thought so that other people can read it….But it's right about there, right about when we sit down to write that story, that things fall apart" [4]. Aspiring leaders should not despair. Like many difficult and important skills, writing becomes easier with daily practice.

The technical complexity of surgical practice has accelerated at an unprecedented pace in the past decade, and non-operative therapy must be integrated with surgical care. Every branch of surgery has examples. Abdominal aortic aneurysms may be treated via laparotomy or endovascularly, depending upon anatomic variability and patient characteristics. The proper treatment of breast cancer requires knowledge of the cell biology of nuclear receptors and angiogenesis in additional to sentinel lymph node biopsy. Care for patients with choledocholithiasis combines endoscopic retrograde cholangiography and laparoscopic cholecystectomy, each applied expertly. As a consequence of these advances, clinical surgery has become increasingly specialized and narrowly focused. Similar forces affect surgical research. Basic investigation advances apace, and so does health services research, but they use fundamentally different techniques. Surgical leaders are called to promote and coordinate diverse surgical specialties and to simultaneously advance surgical knowledge. The ability to do so rests upon openness to novelty and change and a habit of mind that restlessly seeks the stimulation of new ideas. Pasteur noted "Chance only favours the prepared mind." Just so. Leadership belongs to the curious.

A Call to Leadership

For most, the call to leadership does not arrive with a clarion note, a neon sign that flashes LEAD, LEAD, LEAD or some similar epiphany. Rather, the young faculty member establishes a reputation for clinical excellence, or a robust research program, or becomes a valued teacher, and someone asks for help or collaboration or guidance. Someone asks for leadership. And a little voice whispers, "You can do this. You can reach beyond yourself. Maybe you can be a leader." When this happens, the question to be answered is: Do I really want to help and develop others at the expense of myself? For future leaders, the answer must be yes.

Leadership Phenotype

A leadership stereotype has come to dominate American business and political culture. Leaders are characterized as extroverted, assertive, dominating, and often self-aggrandizing. Twentieth century American history provides many examples—General Douglas MacArthur, President Clinton, General Electric chairman Jack Welch to name a few. In her book, Quiet, author Susan Cain contends that these traits may not actually characterize effective leadership. She writes "Contrary to the Harvard Business School model of vocal leadership, the ranks of effective CEOs turns out to be filled with introverts, including Charles Schwab; Bill Gates; Brenda Barnes, CEO of Sara Lee; and James Copeland, former CEO of Deloitte Touche Tohmatsu. 'Among the most effective leaders I have encountered and worked with in half a century,' the management guru Peter Drucker has written, 'some locked themselves in their office and others were ultra-gregarious. Some were quick and impulsive, while others studied the situation and took forever to come to a decision. The one and only personality trait the effective ones I encountered did have in common was something they did *not* have: They had little or no 'charisma' and little use either for the term or what it signifies'" [5].

Leadership is different than authority. The rapid change and uncertainty that characterizes modern surgical practice requires creative risk taking; effective leaders create an environment in which talented people feel safe to take risks. This confidence comes from knowing that the price of failure is not too great, and from being part of a group of like-minded people. Uncertainty requires creativity to resolve unknowns. Leaders must use influence beyond a position of authority because authority alone does not stimulate creativity.

Creativity flourishes in open and inclusive environments, workplaces where diverse faculty are empowered to achieve their best, settings that celebrate the value of diversity. To achieve this goal, organizations must focus on defining core aspects of diversity, examining gaps in diversity and systematic bias, and implementing explicit strategies to improve equality. An ongoing effort to improve cultural competence is key. Cultural competence is the ability to interact effectively with people across different cultures. The components of cultural competence are awareness of one's own cultural worldview (and biases), a positive attitude towards cultural differences, knowledge of different cultural practices, and cross-cultural communication skills. Implicit biases can perpetuate racial and gender disparities in impactful areas such as policy development, hiring, and leadership opportunities. Subtle biases can create an environment in which not everyone is or feels included. By implementing collective strategies to address implicit bias, organizations strengthen both individual faculty members and the collective group.

Achieving workforce diversity requires recruitment of groups currently underrepresented in surgery. The potential benefits of increasing diversity of academic medical faculty have been well-described. Only institutions able to recruit and retain women and underrepresented groups will be likely to maintain the best faculty and house officers.

Leadership Preparation

Many have heard the bromide that "She is a born leader" and have uncritically accepted this truism. Consider an alternative statement that "She is a born surgeon." Almost all surgeons would reject such a notion out of hand. Surgical mastery requires a lifetime of focused work. Surgical training consumes 5–10 years after medical school. Refined physical skills require thousands of hours of intentional practice to obtain and hone; mature judgment is hard earned. According to one study, surgical results improve progressively as surgeons age, peaking in the decade between 50 and 60 years [6]. Surgical mastery surely requires intrinsic talent—physical dexterity, ability to think in three dimensions and concentration—but surgical skill is acquired not intrinsic. That is why it is called the practice of surgery. So too, leadership skills. Potential leaders need to possess relevant talents, including confidence, altruism and analytical ability. Leadership skills are built on this foundation.

Aspiring leaders require additional preparation beyond those experiences described above to function optimally in our complex health care system. For many, enrollment in a formal leadership development program is beneficial. Aspects of leadership preparation programs are covered in detail in other chapters of this volume. The following elements are essential:

1. Leading change
2. Team building
3. Innovation

4. Strategy
5. Finance
6. Marketing
7. Operations management
8. Health care policy.

In 2012, the Department of Surgery at the University of Michigan inaugurated the Leadership Development Program in Surgery. The yearlong program was explicitly designed to include each of the content domains listed, and was directed at Michigan's emerging surgical leaders. The initial class included 24 mid-level faculty members in the Department of Surgery, approximately 20% of total surgical faculty. The Leadership Development Program was led by Dr. Justin Dimick, Associate Chair for Faculty Affairs in the Department of Surgery and by Dr. Christy Lemak, Director of the Griffith Leadership Center and The National Center for Healthcare Leadership within the Michigan School of Public Health. The faculty for the Leadership Development Program was drawn from the Medical School, School of Public Health and the Ross School of Business at the University of Michigan. Being able to draw faculty from three top-ten schools on the same central campus was deemed essential for the success of the program. The program, refined continuously, has now completed its fourth iteration. Fully 62% of Michigan Surgery faculty members have participated in the Leadership Development Program.

For the Leadership Development Program, participants were self-nominated. Leadership development programs intended for medical professionals benefit by having a broad representation of specialties; such diversity is helpful by providing a range of experiences and perspectives. For this program, the participants had each demonstrated personal achievement in clinical care, research and teaching and had made an overt decision to seek broader engagement. Asking potential participants to write an essay outlining their aspirations is a useful way to gauge future goals. Essays were required of participants in the Michigan Leadership Development Program.

Successful leadership development programs boost group morale and create strong teams, but team building takes time. For this to happen, potential participants must fully commit to the time needed and schedules must be rearranged to assure unbroken attendance. The instructional sessions for the Leadership Development Program consisted of a series of all-day Friday blocks. The meetings were held on-campus but remote from the hospital. Prospective participants were required to commit to all sessions and to forego any other activities—clinical work, professional travel, vacation, etc.—for all sessions. Inability to make this commitment precluded participation. Administrative leaders were then contacted to rearrange schedules so that this obligation would be met. Assurances were provided that no financial penalty would apply to any leadership program participant because of absence from other scheduled activities.

Leadership programs must begin with well-articulated visions and goals. The goals of the Michigan Leadership Development Program were to provide emerging leaders with the knowledge, perspectives and tools required to succeed in the contemporary medical environment. These goals were to be met through exposure to thought leaders and content experts in relevant topical fields, through team-building exercises and via self-initiated team-building projects.

Leadership programs are generally benefitted by having practicing leaders provide instruction. For example, health care finance is a topic of every program. Learning how to calculate a return on investment (ROI) or the meaning of net present value (NPV) are crucial exercises. These topics have been covered by professors from the Ross School of Business and the School of Public Health. However, examining a balance sheet detached from real-world context, while crucial, is admittedly also a dry exercise for most clinicians. These topics come to life when the University Hospital CEO follows the didactic session by explaining the long-term sources and uses of hospital capital, and especially when the Department of Surgery chair uses the department's balance sheet as a teaching aid. These topics are typically not widely shared with faculty, but transparency builds trust and helps prepare emerging leaders for future responsibilities.

Many leadership programs entail the performance of projects that seek to build coherent teams and to solve currently pressing problems. These efforts are helpful to illustrate the use of the topics covered in the curriculum, for example, financial analysis or operational optimization. In the Leadership Development Program, the participants were divided into a series of teams, most with four members. Self-selected projects were proposed and then vetted by the entire group. Deliverable outcomes were required. After group approval, funding and personnel resources were provided. Projects ranged from referring physician outreach to creation of new clinical programs to development of unique electronic media for postgraduate teaching.

Formal preparation should be followed by leadership auditions. Every participant in the Leadership Development Program was provided opportunity for a larger leadership role within the Department of Surgery. In any department of surgery there are many opportunities: clerkship director, associate chair for research, division head, residency program director. The auditions were structured to give graded responsibilities and the possibility of larger leadership roles. These tests of leadership were designed to answer two fundamental questions. From the perspectives of the other members of the department: Is the developing leader growing as a leader? From the perspective of the new leader: Am I comfortable and energized by the service of others? And, is this something I want to be a permanent part of my life?

Leadership development is stimulated by feedback. A powerful tool for intermittent feedback is the 360° evaluation method. In this process, differing perspectives of the faculty leader—from supervisors, peers, direct reports, nurses, and house staff—provide appraisal of strengths, weaknesses and areas for improvement. The responses are rendered anonymous to encourage candor. Usually, both a structured evaluation instrument and written comments are provided. All participants in the Leadership Development Program were required to participate in a 360° evaluation. A series of professional coaching sessions followed to first interpret the results and then to suggest methods for leadership improvement.

All leaders need periodic feedback on their performances as leaders. The structure of the 360 method with its holistic view and anonymous evaluations helps leaders see themselves as others see them. Leadership improves with practice. What changes is the leader's capacity to use interpersonal relationships to engage others, and through this engagement, to shape events.

Leading from the Middle

The most effective leaders do not always lead from the front. If a culture is open and inclusive, and if group members are full engaged, transformational leadership comes from the middle.

As Chatman and Kennedy note, "The obvious traits such as confidence, dominance, assertiveness or intelligence, have not, it turns out, shown the level of predictive validity that one would hope for. Rather, we suggest three subtle but likely more powerful qualities that transcend particular individual differences and behaviors. They are a leader's diagnostic capabilities, the breadth and flexibility of his behavioral repertoire, and his understanding of the leadership paradox" [7]. Here diagnostic acumen is meant as the ability to determine for every situation the unique contribution that the leader could make to crafting a solution to that particular circumstance. The obvious value is that every challenge is considered on its own merits and that proposed solutions are tailored. It also follows that leaders need a broad and flexible array of behaviors to respond to an equally wide array of complex situations.

The effective leader is very self-aware, has a clear moral center, is personally balanced, and is interpersonally skilled, but ultimately, is also dispensable. Effective leaders are dispensable because they create a culture of shared decision making and attract other leaders. The most powerful strategy, the hardest to create but the most durable, is creating a culture in which leaders develop other leaders and provide experience which is useful for that purpose. As Chapman and Kennedy observe, "The ultimate test of leadership is how well the team does when the leader is not present" [7]. That is the leadership paradox.

New Leaders

A new generation of surgical leaders is emerging. Their strong surgical leadership will assure that the discipline of Surgery remains at the forefront of contemporary medical practice. Surgical leadership that is imaginative, engaged with other specialties, and open to new ideas will draw the best lessons from the past to build a positive future. This form of leadership, at its best, will motivate departure from the routine, stimulate new learning and inspire new action. Change is everywhere. Creative change requires creative leadership.

References

1. Haynes AB, Weiser TG, Berry WR, et al. A surgical safety checklist to reduce morbidity and mortality in a global population. N Engl J Med. 2009;360:491–9.
2. Porter ME, Nohria N. What is leadership? The CEO's role in large, complex organizations. Brighton, MA: Harvard Business Press; 2010. p. 433–73.
3. Page S. The diversity bonus: how great teams pay off in the knowledge economy. Princeton, NJ: Princeton University Press; 2017.

4. Patchett A. This is the story of a happy marriage. New York: HarperCollins; 2013.
5. Cain S. Quiet. New York: Broadway Books; 2012.
6. Waljee JF, Greenfield LJ, Dimick JB, Birkmeyer JD. Surgeon age and operative mortality in the United States. Ann Surg. 2006;244:353–62.
7. Chatman JA, Kennedy JA. Psychological perspectives on leadership. In: Handbook of leadership theory and practice. Brighton, MA: Harvard Business Press; 2010. p. 159–81.

Leadership Theories and Styles

3

Melina R. Kibbe

Introduction

In order to become an effective leader, one must understand the core leadership theories and the leadership styles that emerged from them, how they evolved, and how to implement different styles of leadership depending on the environment, situation, or need of the leader. Physicians, and more specifically surgeons, are natural leaders as they are accustomed to quick decision-making and tend to be authoritative. However, the very nature of the work of a surgeon can often breed leaders with autocratic leadership styles, a style not conducive to the success of a current day surgical department. Over time, as generational changes have occurred, the traditional autocratic leadership style, so natural to surgeons from the Silent Generation (those born from 1920–1945), no longer resonates well with today's Generation X and Generation Y surgery faculty and trainees. Below, core leadership theories are discussed, followed by a description of some of the common leadership styles that have emerged from the theories. Lastly, a discussion of leadership in surgery with respect to these different leadership styles is presented.

Leadership Theories

Trait Theories

Trait theories argue that effective leaders share common personality traits or characteristics. These include qualities such as integrity, honesty, assertiveness,

M. R. Kibbe (✉)
Department of Surgery, University of North Carolina at Chapel Hill, Chapel Hill, NC, USA

Department of Biomedical Engineering, University of North Carolina at Chapel Hill, Chapel Hill, NC, USA
e-mail: melina_kibbe@med.unc.edu

© Springer Nature Switzerland AG 2019
M. R. Kibbe, H. Chen (eds.), *Leadership in Surgery*, Success in Academic Surgery, https://doi.org/10.1007/978-3-030-19854-1_3

decisiveness, motivation, innovation, vision, intelligence, persuasion, etc. Early trait theories posed that leadership traits are innate and that one is born to be a leader. Trait theories have now evolved and pose that leadership traits can be learned, and that positive leadership traits can be developed through training and education. Many studies on leadership traits have been conducted in an attempt to identify traits of successful leaders. The Forbes list of top ten qualities that make a great leader include: honesty, creativity, intuition, confidence, commitment, ability to inspire, delegate, and communicate, a sense of humor, and positive attitude [1]. While many of the above traits are associated with great leaders, it should be noted that the converse does not necessarily hold true, i.e. that those who possess these traits, or a combination of these traits guarantees that one will be a successful leader. Chapter 4 in this textbook explores leadership trait theories in-depth as well as some of the common traits of successful leaders.

Behavioral Theories

Behavioral theories focus on how a leader behaves. In the early 1930s, Kurt Lewin presented a framework based on the behaviors of leaders [2]. He described three types of leadership behaviors: (1) autocratic; (2) democratic; and (3) laissez-faire. Autocratic leaders are described as making autonomous decisions with no consultation amongst their team members. This type of leadership is appropriate when quick decisions need to be made, when there is no need for consensus, or when consensus from the team is not necessary in order for a successful outcome to be achieved. Conversely, Democratic leaders do take into consideration input from the team before making a decision. The degree of input considered will vary from leader to leader. This type of leadership is appropriate when team consensus is important for the final outcome. However, this style of leadership can be difficult to manage when a wide variety of opinions, perspectives, and ideas exist among the team members. Finally, Laissez-faire leaders typically do not interfere with the decision-making process. These leaders allow the individuals in the team to make most of the decisions. This type of leadership is appropriate when the teams consist of highly competent, skilled, motivated and capable individuals that require little supervision. This leadership style can fail when it is born out of laziness on the part of the leader. Since the description of these three leadership styles, many more styles have emerged. A description of the most common leadership styles follows below.

Contingency or Situational Theories

Contingency or situational leadership theories pose that no one leadership style is the correct style. Instead, the best leadership style is the one dictated by the situation or circumstance (i.e., situational leadership). For example, if a quick decision is required, the autocratic leadership style might be best. If the full support of all team members is required, the democratic leadership style might be best. Contingent leadership theories also pose that the best leadership style depends on characteristics of the team members. For instance, the Hersey-Blanchard Situational Leadership Theory proposes that successful leaders should change their leadership styles based on the maturity of the people on the team and the details of the task [3]. Hersey and Blanchard describe four leadership styles for this theory (i.e., telling, selling, participating, and delegating) and four maturity levels. The use of each style is dictated by the maturity level of the team members. If the team members have a low maturity, the telling style works best. If the team members have high maturity, the delegating style works best. Another leadership model, the Dunham and Pierce Leadership Process Model, describes how four factors contribute to leadership success or failure [4]. These factors are: the leader, the followers, the context, and the outcome. All four variables are related to each other and affect each other. This model highlights that leadership is dynamic and that it is important to be flexible based on the context, the outcome, and the team.

Power and Influence Theories

Power and influence theories are based on the different ways in which leaders use their power and influence to get things done. These theories then examine the leadership styles that emerge as a result. For example, powerful people gravitate towards leadership and therefore are followed by others, but there are often different reasons why people have power. One of the best-known theories that describes this type of leadership is French and Raven's Five Forms of Power [5]. John French and Bertram Raven described five forms of power: legitimate, reward, expert, referent, and coercive. Legitimate power comes from the belief that that person has the right to make demands and expect compliance, such as a CEO or president. Reward power is when someone has the power to compensate others for their actions (i.e., salary increase, bonus, etc.). Expert power comes from a person's own superior skill or knowledge (i.e., recognized expertise). Referent power results from a person's perceived worthiness, charm, charisma, or appeal, often apparent in celebrities, or some politicians. Coercive power results when someone has the ability to punish others. When a person recognizes their source of power they are better able to lead for the best outcome. The positional power sources (i.e., legitimate, reward, and coercive) tend to be the least effective as they can easily fail, as workers feel they themselves have no power or are not emotionally vested to follow these leaders. Personal power sources (i.e., expert and referent) tend to be the most effective, as leaders with these qualities often tend to be more motivating and interpersonal when dealing with workers.

Emotional Intelligence

Emotional intelligence is the ability to understand and manage your emotions as well as handle interpersonal relationships with the people around you (direct reports, peers, and supervisors). Leaders with high emotional intelligence are able to remain calm, control their tempers and manage a crisis with great skill. They are able to recognize their own emotions, what these emotions mean, how these emotions can influence others, and are then able to modulate their leadership style based on this information. Having emotional intelligence is essential for a leader. First popularized by Daniel Goleman, five elements of emotional intelligence have been described: (1) self-awareness; (2) self-regulation; (3) motivation; (4) empathy; and (5) social skills [6]. The more a leader is able to understand how their emotions and actions impact others and is able to manage each of these five elements, the higher the emotional intelligence. The higher the emotional intelligence, the more successful he or she will be as a leader, as they are able to relate to and work more productively with others. To learn more about emotional intelligence and these five elements, the reader is directed to Chap. 5 on emotional intelligence.

Leadership Styles

Many different leadership styles have been born from the core leadership theories described previously. A brief description of some of the more common leadership styles is provided.

Autocratic Leadership

As described previously, autocratic leadership is characterized by a leader who makes decisions with very little input from others. Autocratic leaders tend to have a lot of power over the people they lead. A benefit of this type of leadership is that it is very efficient in certain situations. It is an appropriate leadership tactic when quick decisions need to be made, when there is no need for consensus, or when consensus from the team is not necessary in order for a successful outcome to be achieved. This type of leadership works well in crises where quick decisions must be made and followed (i.e., trauma bay or operating room). It works well for the military as it allows the troops to focus their attention and energy on performing the task at hand. It also works well for jobs that require routine tasks or involve unskilled labor. A disadvantage to this type of leadership is that many people resent having no input or no sense of ownership in their work environment. It can result in high levels of job dissatisfaction and turnover. Autocratic leadership is an extreme form of transactional leadership, which will be discussed later.

Democratic or Participative Leadership

Democratic leaders include the team members in the decision-making process, but ultimately make the final decisions themselves. Democratic leaders encourage creativity, participation, and input from the team members. As a result, team members feel a greater sense of purpose toward the common mission and tend to be very engaged in the project, work and/or decision, and hence more productive. Benefits of democratic leadership are many and include high job satisfaction among the team members and greater motivation of the workers since they feel a sense of inclusion, empowerment, and ownership within the decision-making process. This type of leadership also tends to result in greater development of the skills of the team members, supporting even more engagement. This leadership style is most suitable for situations in which working as a team is necessary, and when quality is more important than productivity or efficiency. However, a distinct disadvantage of this type of leadership is that it takes time to make and execute decisions, especially compared to autocratic leadership. Thus, it can hinder speed and efficiency and would not be ideal during times of crisis. Lastly, this type of leadership only works well when the team members have the knowledge and/or expertise to contribute meaningfully to the decision-making process.

Bureaucratic Leadership

Bureaucratic leaders are rule followers and work "by the book". They ensure that everyone follows the rules and procedures rigorously and precisely. Advantages of this leadership style are precision, efficiency, and predictable output. This style of leadership functions well for tasks that require a high degree of accuracy and safety, such as operating heavy machinery, working with caustic or explosive chemicals, or at extreme heights. It works well for jobs that handle large amounts of currency, such as cashiers, currency exchange personnel, and bankers. It is also ideal for activities that are very routine, such as manufacturing. Disadvantages of this leadership style are that creativity and innovation are stifled because of the rigid, inflexible framework. It can also create resentment among the team members if the leader obtains the position because of conformity and rule following and not because of qualifications or recognized expertise.

Charismatic Leadership

Charismatic leaders inspire enthusiasm in their team members and are often engaging and energetic, thus motivating others to excel. The ability to create excitement and commitment among the team members has great benefit. In a way, this type of leadership can resemble transformational leadership which will be is discussed later. However, the main distinction between charismatic leadership and transformational leadership lies with the intent of the leader. Transformational leaders want to inspire change in their team members or organization. Charismatic leaders are often inwardly focused and do not necessarily want to lead change. This can be a disadvantage as they can be more interested in themselves than their team members or organization. Charismatic leaders also have a sense of superiority and often do not accept criticism well, but due to their heightened sense of self-worth, charismatic leaders are often viewed as successful by their team members. From an organizational point of view, if a charismatic leader suddenly departs there is often a great risk that the project, team, or organization will collapse given the inherent focus on the leader and not the team or organization.

Laissez-Faire Leadership

As discussed previously, laissez-faire leaders, (also known as passive-avoidant leaders), typically do not interfere with the decision-making process. These leaders allow the individuals in the team to make most of the decisions. They typically allow the team members complete freedom to do their work when and how they like, including setting their own deadlines. This type of leadership works best when the teams consist of highly competent, skilled, motivated, and capable individuals who require very little supervision. This leadership style also works well when the leaders monitor performance and provide regular feedback. One of the main advantages of this leadership style is that team members tend to have very high job satisfaction and productivity given the autonomy they are permitted. A disadvantage of this type of leadership style is when it emerges out of laziness on the part of the leader. In addition, this type of leadership style fails if the team members are not internally motivated, or don't have the skill or knowledge to do their jobs. Finally, a laissez-faire leader can downplay concerns or issues that the team might be experiencing and avoid conflict or mediation, taking the more "hands-off" approach to leadership.

People-Oriented or Relations-Oriented Leadership

People- or relations-oriented leaders are completely focused on developing, organizing, and supporting the people on the team. This leadership style requires participation and teamwork, and tends to support creativity and collaborations. People-oriented leaders tend to treat everyone on the team equally. They are usually very approachable and friendly leaders, and pay close attention to the welfare of all the team members. These leaders are also readily available in times of need by any team member. An advantage of this style of leadership is that people enjoy being on teams with people-oriented leaders. Team members led in this way tend to be productive and are more willing to take risks because they know the leader will support them if they need it. This leadership style tends to be the opposite of task-oriented leadership which is discussed below. A disadvantage of this leadership style is when the leader goes too far and prioritizes the development of the team above the task, project, or organization.

Task-Oriented Leadership

Task-oriented leaders focus on getting the task or job done. These leaders share some traits with autocratic and bureaucratic leaders. Task-oriented leaders begin by defining the work to be done, and the roles required of the team members. They then put structure in place to complete the task, including the planning and organization of how the work will proceed, and finally, monitor the output. These leaders are excellent at creating and maintaining performance standards. An advantage of this style of leadership is that tasks are often completed in a timely manner. This style is also helpful for team members who need lots of direction and do not manage their time wisely. Disadvantages of this leadership style are low job satisfaction and morale due to lack of ownership over projects, which can lead to high turnover with low retention rates among team members.

Servant Leadership

A servant leader is someone who leads by simply meeting the needs of the team at large. They often don't recognize themselves as the leader and serve in this capacity more out of duty and by leading through example. Servant leaders tend to stay away from the limelight and glory of leading. They prefer to get the work done and have the team receive the recognition, not themselves as leaders. Given these characteristics, these leaders tend to have very high integrity and generosity. Servant leadership is a form of democratic leadership since the entire team is involved in the decision-making process. This type of leadership is useful for tasks or projects that place emphasis on values. In fact, servant leaders tend to move up the ladder based on their values. Under the power and influence theory, this would be most similar to expert power, as servant leaders gain power because of their values, ideals, and ethics in addition to knowledge, skills and expertise. Servant leadership also tends to create a positive team and corporate attitude with high morale. A disadvantage of servant leadership is the time required to master this type of leadership, and the time required to complete tasks and projects. Similar to democratic leadership, it can take a lot of time for the team members to make decisions. Thus, this leadership style is less conducive for situations that require quick decisions or have tight deadlines. Another disadvantage of this leadership style relates to competitive leadership positions. Servant leaders tend to trail behind leaders using other styles in competitive situations.

Transactional Leadership

Transactional leadership implies that a worker or team member is paid or compensated in some manner for their work product or services (i.e., a transaction). If the work is not done, the leader has the right to be punitive. Thus, team members are motivated by reward and punishment, and transactional leadership can be described as having two components: (1) contingent reward and (2) management by exception. This style of leadership is similar to having coercive power as the source of power described from the power and influence theories. An advantage of this type of leadership is that roles and responsibilities are clearly delineated. People with great ambition tend to excel with this type of leadership since performance is evaluated solely on the accomplishments of the individual and not the team.

A disadvantage of this leadership style is the potential for low job satisfaction. Team members can do little to change their job situation which can lead to high employee turnover. This type of leadership is typical of managerial positions. It is not conducive to situations that require creativity and innovation. Some would argue that this is not a leadership style at all, as the focus is on task completion. However, others argue that this leadership style is similar to task-oriented leadership.

Transformational Leadership

Transformational leaders inspire workers and team members with a shared vision of the future. It is a vision that is usually ambitious yet rich, exciting, and attainable. Transformational leaders set clear goals, inspire people to work toward those goals, and manage delivery of the vision. These leaders also coach and develop the team members by recognizing the potential of their team members and engaging them intellectually to achieve their full potential. They provide regular feedback and serve as good mentors. Transformational leaders also tend to have very high integrity and outstanding communication skills. Given all of these attributes, transformational leadership has been described as having four components: (1) idealized influence; (2) inspirational motivation; (3) intellectual stimulation; and (4) individualized consideration. Currently, this is one of the most successful types of leadership in the business world. An advantage of this type of leadership is that because these leaders tend to expect the very best of the team members, team members are highly satisfied, productive, and engaged. Thus, job turnover is lower compared to other types of leadership. A disadvantage of this type of leadership is inherently linked to the enthusiasm of the leader—they tend to need support from the detail people. This is why one often observes transformational leaders being supported by transactional leaders (i.e., the managers), with the latter being the individuals who complete the work.

Adaptive Leadership

Adaptive leaders employ several of the leadership styles described above. The role of an adaptive leader is to guide the team members through problem solving. Adaptive leaders engage the team members, empower and motivate them to solve the adaptive problem on their own. This process requires thoughtful direction on the part of the leader. An advantage of this style of leadership is that any change is more likely to be sustainable than if it were decreed from an autocratic leadership style. The latter type of change is usually transient. This type of leadership style is good for organizations in need of culture change. A disadvantage of this style of leadership is that it can take time for the team members to solve the problem. This leadership style also requires that the team members have some knowledge, skill, and expertise with the problem being addressed. This strategy can be helpful in the health care industry when physicians are leading physicians and the desire is a sustainable culture change.

Leadership in Surgery

No one leadership style is right for everyone. Surgeons by nature, and due to our training paradigm, tend to exhibit autocratic, task-oriented, and transactional leadership styles. However, there are times when democratic, bureaucratic, servant, and definitely transformational leadership is required. Due to this, some would argue that situational leadership is the best theory to expound, as it takes into account the needs of the team members, the organization, and tasks in determining the best leadership style that fits those needs. For example, in the operating room, a democratic team approach is needed between the anesthetists, nursing staff, and surgeons. However, in times of crisis, an autocratic style clearly works best. Similarly, in the clinics, a collaborative democratic approach is required between the scheduling clerks, nurses, and physicians. But, when it comes to managing a specific ailment, disease, or complication, the physician will need to take charge and be decisive. For a Chair of a Department of Surgery, depending on the needs of the institution and the need for change management, a transformational leadership style may work best. When consensus is needed, a democratic approach is helpful. Yet, surgeons also still require some form of transactional leadership in the sense of reward and punishment. The later especially applies to matters of compensation.

Many studies have been conducted examining leadership styles in the health care industry. Xirasagar et al. [7] surveyed executive directors of community health care centers using a Likert-type scale. They found that transformational leadership was used most often. The executives found it most effective and felt that it resulted in the greatest subordinate satisfaction and effort. Transactional leadership closely followed transformational leadership, and laissez-faire leadership trailed a distant third. An examination of rural primary care physicians by Hana and Kirkhaug revealed that physicians used change style leadership (i.e., transformational) the most, followed by task style (i.e., task-oriented), and then relation style [8]. Interestingly, lead physicians were noted to use mostly change style, whereas age was negatively correlated with the use of change and relation style. A survey of physician medical and executive directors of health care systems also revealed the highest scores for transformational leadership as compared to transactional and laissez-faire [9]. A similar survey of deans of nursing programs showed that 77% of the deans scored highest with transformational leadership, 21% for transactional leadership, and 2% for passive-avoidant leadership [10]. Thus, it is clear that a good leader should be well-versed in the different styles of leadership and use them appropriately, as dictated by the need.

Conclusion

Several different leadership core theories exist. These theories have evolved over time but take into account leadership traits, leadership behavior, the situation (i.e., contingency theory), the source of power and influence, and emotional intelligence. From these, many leadership styles have emerged to describe how leaders function to achieve a successful outcome. These styles include autocratic, democratic, bureaucratic, charismatic, laissez-faire, people or relations-oriented, task-oriented, servant, transactional, transformational, and adaptive leadership. No one leadership style is right for one person or one situation. However, studies on leadership in the health care arena reveal that the most effective leaders have adopted a significant portion of their leadership style as transformational, a style very popular in the business world. Varying contributions of other styles also comprise a good leader's armamentarium and it is important to understand when one style is better over another. Surgeons are uniquely positioned to be leaders. However, it is imperative that surgeons recognize that their training paradigm has a tendency to produce an autocratic leadership style, a style rarely effective in the health care industry. Through education and training about the various leadership theories and styles, a surgeon can be well-positioned to lead.

References

1. Prive T. Top 10 qualities that make a great leader; 12/19/2012; Forbes http://www.forbes.com/sites/tanyaprive/2012/12/19/top-10-qualities-that-make-a-great-leader/. Accessed 25 June 2014.
2. Lewin K, Lippitt R, White RK. Patterns of aggressive behavior in experimentally created social climates. J Soc Psychol. 1939;10:271–301.
3. Hersey P, Blanchard KH, Johnson DE. Management of organizational behavior: utilizing human resources. 7th ed. Upper Saddle River, NJ: Prentice Hall; 1996. p. 188–223.
4. Pierce JL, Dunham RB. Managing. Scott Foresman & Co.: Chicago, IL; 1990.
5. French JRP Jr, Raven BH. The bases of social power. In: Cartwright D, editor. Studies in social power. Ann Arbor, MI: Institute for Social Research; 1959. p. 150–67.
6. Goleman D. Leadership that gets results. Harv Bus Rev. March 2000:78–90.
7. Xirasagar S, Samuels ME, Stoskopf CH. Physician leadership styles and effectiveness: an empirical study. Med Care Res Rev. 2005;62(6):720–40.
8. Hana J, Kirkhaug R. Physicians' leadership styles in rural primary medical care: how are they perceived by staff? Scand J Prim Health Care. 2014;32:4–10.
9. Xirasagar S, Samuels ME, Curtin TF. Management training of physician executives, their leadership style, and care management performance: an empirical study. 2/1/2006, AJMC http://www.ajmc.com/publications/issue/2006/2006-02-vol12-n2/feb06-2252p101-108. Accessed 16 June 2014.
10. Broome ME. Self-reported leadership styles of deans of baccalaureate and higher degree nursing programs in the United States. J Prof Nurs. 2013;29(6):323–9.

Are People Born to Lead?

Mary T. Killackey

Introduction

Are leaders born or made? This is one of the most frequently asked questions when discussing leadership development. A Google Scholar search on this topic provided over 1.6 million results with early references attributed to Plato and Machiavelli [1]. Not surprisingly, the answer is not black and white but an amalgam of varying thoughts often not evidence based. Over 100 years of leadership research have led to competing paradigms and no consensus; the debate continues today [2]. The psychologist Warren Bennis wrote in 1959, "….probably more has been written and less is known about leadership than about any other topic in the behavioral sciences" [2, 3]. In a recent Harvard Business Review article, the author puts forth whether the question's focus should be clarified to determine the origins of an *effective* leader [4]. Despite the lack of a clear answer, this question is relevant as one contemplates future career goals and formulates a plan to achieve them.

Background

In an earlier edition of this chapter, Jeffrey Matthews MD provided a comprehensive review of the historical references of the nature versus nurture argument. Early on, the assumption was that leaders were born and the "great man" theory prevailed until the mid-twentieth century. First described in the nineteenth century by Thomas Carlyle, the "great man theory" contends that the qualities necessary for leadership are inherited and most often found in the upper class [5, 6]. As such, "the course of history was determined by the actions of a small number of extraordinary men possessing extraordinary skills" [7]. Following this, the leadership trait theory came into favor, with a focus on identifying

M. T. Killackey (✉)
Department of Surgery, Tulane University School of Medicine, New Orleans, LA, USA
e-mail: mkillack@tulane.edu

© Springer Nature Switzerland AG 2019
M. R. Kibbe, H. Chen (eds.), *Leadership in Surgery*, Success in Academic Surgery, https://doi.org/10.1007/978-3-030-19854-1_4

personality characteristics, motives and behaviors that differentiated leaders from non-leaders, regardless of being inherited or acquired [8]. Gordon Allport concluded that successful leaders have the right combination of traits [5, 9]. A sound scientific method was lacking in the scholarly approach to these theories and their subjects were positional leaders (occupying a leadership position based on pedigree and "right") and not necessarily effective leaders. The complexity of this topic makes it quite difficult to define leadership and without a consensus, research is unreliable. Until recently, most research did not utilize more rigorous scientific methods such as longitudinal evaluations and measurement of outcomes at multiple levels [10]. Eventually, the leadership trait theory fell out of favor as it was clear that possessing specific traits did not alone create a leader.

In the latter half of the twentieth century, behavioral psychologists led the way in defining emergent leadership as it addressed the concern above that leadership traits are situation or context-dependent. The belief was that leaders can be made, and that individuals can learn to become leaders through teaching and observation [5, 11, 12]. As Fielder describes, it is when individuals, possessing the right degree of visibility and the right combination of skills and resources that matched the needs or goals of a group, emerge as acceptable leaders [13]. This contingency theory asserts that leaders come forward when in "the right place at the right time" and there are no universal set of traits a leader must possess. Other conceptual models including transformational leadership and adaptive theory emerged, addressing the transactional nature of leadership [5, 14, 15]. More recently, leadership scholars have gone back around to earlier ideas and are studying traits within the situational context of the relationship between leader and follower.

Current Thought

In an attempt to answer whether there is a leadership gene, DeNeve performed twin studies based on leadership role occupancy [16]. The longitudinal methods indicate an association with rs4950, a single nucleotide polymorphism (SNP) on a neuronal acetylcholine receptor gene: CHRNB3. Similar to earlier twin studies, the results suggest that the heritability of leadership role occupancy is close to one-third while the remaining variance is associated with environmental influences [17, 18]. Some individuals will have a genetic advantage ("good genes") as relates to assuming leadership-related roles, however the results suggest that anyone might become a better leader and with learning and experience, positively influence their opportunity to hold a leadership role. The topic of leadership development effectiveness is just as complex whether leaders are born or made, and also requires more rigorous scientific investigation. What is clear, however, is that within the business world where between 20–40 billion dollars are spent annually on development programs, our actions support the belief that leaders can be made. Furthermore, 86% of respondents to a 2014 survey of business leaders around the world rated broadening, deepening and accelerating leadership development as urgent or important [19, 20].

Interestingly, The less rigorous investigations into the born versus made question have led to similar conclusions. In 2012, the Center for Creative Leadership (CCL) published the results of a survey given to top executives, specifically asking whether leaders were born or made [21]. Just over half believed leaders are made while 20%

believe leaders are born with inherent traits. Almost 30% felt that both are important. When each group was asked to prioritize specific development elements: training, experiences or traits, the "Born" cohort chose traits (41%) in comparison to the "Made" group, which chose experiences (45.6%) followed closely by training (34.45%). Interestingly, the "Born" group also highly valued experiences (38.23%). The authors suggest that the difference may actually be seen in the behavior of each group. The "Born" group may be selective in who gets the development "experiences" whereas the "Made" group may be more inclusive in offering experience opportunities.

The CCL points out that there is value in understanding the beliefs of those in top-level leadership roles as it may influence recruitment, promotion and the investment into leader development programs. Believers of the born theory may focus on selection (identify the "right" people) as compared to the made theory, where the emphasis is on ensuring the people you have are given the right opportunities to develop into leaders. Understanding the leaders' beliefs may also lead to behavior adaptation, not only to ensure tasks are achieved but also to assess our likelihood to obtain leadership roles that we may be seeking. "Top leaders set the tone for the development of others within their organization, so understanding their view" can help you understand your own opportunities for leadership [21].

A 2005 Harvard Business Review article describes the 25 year experience studying more than 6000 business executives and further supports the benefit of a focused approach to developing leadership skills [22, 23]. Measuring leadership actions using well-described performance parameters, the authors conclude that those individuals with the willingness to be self-reflective and develop themselves can successfully advance along the continuum of leadership development profiles (Table 4.1). More importantly, institutions that commit to prioritizing leadership development may economically transform their companies.

Table 4.1 Seven types of action logics [24]

Leadership profile	Description	Skill level	% cohort
Opportunist	Tendency to focus on personal wins, sees world/people as opportunities to be exploited	Below average	5
Diplomat	Loyally serves group, seeks to please higher status colleagues while avoid/ignore conflict		12
Expert	Exercises control by perfecting their knowledge; pursues continuous improvement and considers emotional intelligence as irrelevant		38
Achiever	Creates positive work environment, focus on deliverables may inhibit thinking outside the box	Average	30
Individualist	Puts personalities and ways of relating into perspective as is aware of potential conflict between principles and actions; may ignore rules deemed irrelevant	Above average	10
Strategist	Treats organizational constraints as transformable; adept at creating shared visions that encourage individual and organizational transformations		4
Alchemist	Ability to renew or reinvent themselves and their organizations in historically significant ways; has capacity to deal simultaneously with many situations at multiple levels without losing sight of long-term goals	Rare	1

Are Surgeons Born or Made?

Beginning with the assumption that surgeons are leaders, the literature is sparse in addressing this question. While most would agree that surgeons have at the least, an affinity for leadership and a willingness to take on significant responsibility, it does not automatically translate into effective leadership. Traditionally surgeons have expressed an authoritative style of leadership that may have been more "natural". The current emphasis in surgical leadership has shifted from the traditional autocratic and transactional styles to a more transformational model [24]. Modern leadership styles for surgeons now require additional training, development and enhancement of skills—thus made [5, 25]. While technical competence and clinical acumen are essential, successful surgeon leaders will exemplify:

- Professionalism (adhere to and model ethical principles, take responsibility for actions),
- Motivation (desire and energy directed to achieving a goal),
- Innovation (open to new ideas, embrace change, exhibit creativity),
- Resilience (optimism, the capacity to recover from setbacks, forge a new course),
- Teamwork (form an effective, diverse team with common goal, shared responsibility),
- Communication skills (convey important information so that it is received, in multimodal fashion—not just facts but overall strategic vision and purpose),
- Business acumen (essential management skills, transparency, transactional understanding),
- Effective teaching (ability to teach knowledge, develop leadership team) and
- Emotional intelligence (humility, empathy, self-awareness, self-regulation).

While surgeons may hold some or all of the traits associated with these skills, surgeon leaders must invest the time to further develop themselves as well as those under their supervision. A 2013 review of the development of surgical experts acknowledges that technical skill is at the core of surgical training and some individuals may have innate capabilities making it easier to develop these skills [26]. The authors highlight a study performed in the UK which studied medical students' introduction to arthroscopic procedures. They classified the novices into three groups of surgical ability: innately gifted almost from the outset, able to reach competency with repeated practice on simulator and those who could not achieve basic competency despite repeated practice. Does this hold true for leadership ability? The authors recognized the lack of research in the development of non-technical skills among surgeons and advocated for further exploration as it will be essential for the development of effective surgical training programs. The authors conclude that while some individuals possess innate abilities that set them apart from the rest, surgical experts are made and not born. Not surprisingly, due to the lack of hard evidence for the right balance and form of non-technical skills training, many surgical programs are just starting to incorporate such curricula. For those surgeons already in practice, myriad leader development programs have begun to address this need. Mentorship, coaching, networking and 360° evaluations all have their role in the making of a leader as well. There is not nor will there be a consensus on the best or right way to develop leadership skills, as each individual's needs are unique.

In summary, the adage that someone is "born to lead" has its place in historical reference but does not sufficiently acknowledge the question of whether leaders are born or made. Despite the vast number of writings, most are not evidence based and fell out of fashion at a particular point. Current psychologists are now employing more rigorous scientific methods to this research arena—most importantly, longitudinal studies that will address leader effectiveness rather than just leader role occupancy. These studies should enhance the few heritability studies which produced the generally accepted rate of about 1/3 of leadership as inherited in some way. In the meantime, we will have to be content with the moderate view that the answer is both—a hopeful position for anyone wanting to be a leader in surgery.

References

1. https://scholar.google.com/scholar?hl=en&as_sdt=0%2C10&q=are+leaders+born+or+made&oq=are+leaders.
2. Antonakis J, Day D, editors. The nature of leadership. 3rd ed. Thousand Oaks, CA: Sage Publications, Inc.; 2018. p. 4.
3. Bennis W. Leadership theory and administrative behavior: the problem of authority. Adm Sci Q. 1959;4(3):259–301.
4. Locke C. Asking whether leaders are born or made is the wrong question. Harv Bus Rev. 2014. https://hbr.org/2014/03/asking-whether-leaders-are-born-or-made-is-the-wrong-question.
5. Patel V, Warren O, Humphris P, et al. What does leadership in surgery entail? ANZ J Surg. 2010;80(12):876–83.
6. Carlyle T. Lectures on heroes, hero-worship and the heroic in history. Nebraska: University of Nebraska Press; 1841.
7. Zaccaro S. Trait-based perspectives of leadership. Am Psychol. 2007;62:6–16.
8. Kirkpatrick S, Locke E. Leadership: do traits matter? Executive. 1991;5:48–60.
9. Allport F, Allport G. Personality traits: their classification and measurement. J Abnorm Soc Psychol. 1921;16:1–40.
10. Day D, Thornton A. Leadership development. In: Antonakis J, Day D, editors. The nature of leadership. 3rd ed. Thousand Oaks, CA: Sage Publications, Inc.; 2018. p. 356.
11. McGregor D. Human side of enterprise. New York: McGraw-Hill; 1960.
12. Blake R, Mouton J. The managerial grid: the key to leadership excellence. Houston: Gulf Publishing Company; 1964.
13. Fielder D. Research on leadership selection and training: one view of the future. Adm Sci Q. 1996;41:241–50.
14. Burns J. Leadership. New York: Harper & Row; 1978.
15. Heifetz R. Leadership without easy answers. Cambridge, MA: Belknap Press of Harvard University Press; 1994.
16. DeNeve J, Mikhaylov S, Dawes C, et al. Born to lead? A twin design and genetic association study of leadership role occupancy. Leadersh Q. 2013;24:45–60.
17. Arvey R, Rotundo M, Johnson W, et al. The determinants of leadership role occupancy: genetic and personality factors. Leadersh Q. 2006;17:1–20.
18. Zhang Z, Ilies R, Arvey R. Beyond genetic explanations for leadership: the moderating role of the social environment. Organ Behav Hum Decis Process. 2009;110:118–28.
19. Lamoureux K. High-impact leadership development: best practices, vendor profiles and industry solutions. Oakland, CA: Bersin and Associates; 2007.

20. O'Leonard K, Krider J. Leadership development factbook 2014: benchmarks and trends in US leadership development. Oakland, CA: Bersin and Associates; 2014.
21. Gentry W, Deal J, Stawiski S, et al. Are leaders born or made? Perspectives from the executive suite: Center for Creative Leadership; 2012. p. 4–6.
22. Buchler P, Martin D, Knaebel H, et al. Leadership characteristics and business management of modern academic surgery. Langenbecks Arch Surg. 2006;391(2):149–56.
23. Rooke D, Torbert W. 7 transformations of leadership. Harv Bus Rev. 2005;83(4):66–76.
24. Prabhakaran S, Economopoulos K, Grabo D, et al. Surgical leadership across generations. The Bulletin, American College of Surgeons. 2012.
25. Souba W. Leadership and strategic alignment-getting people on board and engaged. J Surg Res. 2001;96:144–51.
26. Sadideen H, Alvand A, Saadeddin, et al. Surgical experts: born or made? Int J Surg. 2013;11:773–8.

Understanding Emotional Intelligence and Its Role in Leadership

5

Harry C. Sax and Bruce L. Gewertz

Introduction

Irrespective of our life paths, the ability to initiate and sustain effective interactions with others is a key determinant of success and fulfillment. As health care professionals, we must lead in a variety of roles - in hospitals, clinics, operating theatres and increasing, the C Suite. We are often challenged by the stresses of practice and the need to achieve balance with family and friends. Since conflicts occur on a regular basis, a level of personal insight is vital to a healthy and productive life.

The increased interest in emotional intelligence is supported by data demonstrating that enhanced social interactions improve personal performance in a wide range of settings. Boyatzis studied 2000 supervisors and executives and found that 14 of 16 distinguishing traits for success were emotional, not cognitive [1]. Spencer and Spencer defined job competencies in 286 organizations and noted that 18 of 21 competencies associated with high performance were emotionally based [2]. Comparing "star" performers to average performers in diverse industries, Goleman found that emotional advantages were noted twice as frequently in high performers and were a much better predictor of achievement than cognitive superiority [3]. In the recruitment process for academic department chair, Clavien and Deiss emphasize the importance of strong emotional, personal and social skills over other qualifications such as an MBA. Further they found that those with high levels of insight and purpose can inspire others to further their mission and be more resilient to administrative burdens [4]. in other settings, high levels of emotional intelligence among nursing leaders was associated with greater job satisfaction and lower turnover among those they supervise [5, 6] EQ development and nurturing is now being recognized as a vital component of graduate medical education curriculums [7].

H. C. Sax · B. L. Gewertz (✉)
Department of Surgery, Cedars-Sinai Medical Center, Los Angeles, CA, USA
e-mail: Harry.Sax@cshs.org; Bruce.Gewertz@cshs.org

© Springer Nature Switzerland AG 2019
M. R. Kibbe, H. Chen (eds.), *Leadership in Surgery*, Success in Academic Surgery, https://doi.org/10.1007/978-3-030-19854-1_5

In this chapter we will quantify the traits associated with emotional intelligence (EQ), examine the role of EQ in the medical environment, including the differences seen in surgeons, provide insights into the neurobiology of human emotion, address how experiences shape our ability to interact with others, describe how emotional intelligence can be measured and quantified, and finally assess what one can do to improve EQ. We will explore the role of emotional intelligence in conflict resolution and describe forms of feedback that can increase insight and enhance both professional performance and personal satisfaction.

The Scope of Emotional Intelligence

The term "emotional intelligence" describes a set of personal attributes which enhance social and professional relationships. As developed by Goleman and others, these elements span the full range of interactions between individuals and society including self-awareness, self-regulation, social awareness, and relationship management [8, 9].

Self-awareness encompasses one's openness to their own emotional experience and their ability to realistically appraise their skills and abilities and to integrate feedback for self-improvement. It involves a developed ability to see our emotions from some perspective or "distance"—to recognize that we are feeling anger, frustration, unbridled joy, or sorrow. It then allows us not to react immediately to those emotions (Goleman uses the term "hijacking") [8]. Within brief, self-regulation helps us remain above the fray.

This is particularly relevant to surgical practice. Surgeons are trained to have control over their emotions to deal with high stakes situations. As a consequence, we are occasionally unclear of or ignore what we are truly feeling. Under ideal circumstances, there is a proper balance between control and emotion; such an equilibrium would engender appropriate levels of confidence and self-esteem and allow identification of "triggers" that lead to impulsive, negative reactions.

Self-regulation is closely related to self-awareness and is the ability to manage emotions within the context of any situation. Self-regulation is about homeostasis. It is not appropriate to suppress all emotion any more than it is to be carried away into paralyzing dark depths of depression or the dizzying heights of mania. Although it is possible to have strong self-regulation without self-awareness, it is not comfortable and is analogous to addicts who "white knuckle" their way through temptation.

As surgeons and leaders, we cycle through emotions throughout the day. Those with strong self-management are adaptable and are more capable of organizing thoughts and actions. They exhibit high levels of integrity. They remain optimistic in the face of failure and rejection, viewing the setback as additional data on which to set a future course. In contrast, lack of self-regulation results in impulsive responses to a situation, driven by anger or strong emotion. This cycle has derailed many careers.

Social awareness behaviors include empathy, political acumen, organizational dynamics, and openness to opposing points of view. We are social animals, characterized by the need to interact with others. While we can appreciate how we may be feeling in the moment, our deeply held feelings are not always expressed verbally. Up to 85% of communication comes from nonverbal cues—facial expression, tone of voice, subtle body language [8, 10]. The ability to read these cues predicts success in human interaction.

This level of attunement ideally begins in childhood by parents who can mirror their children's feelings, creating an understanding of empathy. Throughout life, however, relationships provide new opportunities to learn empathy, nonverbal communication, and read situations. Those with strong skills in social awareness are seen as good "listeners," demonstrating the ability to understand others' thoughts, feelings and motivations by picking up all the cues.

The final competency is the ability to **manage relationships** despite the normal differences of opinions and conflict that exists within groups. It is not only having the social awareness to read the nonverbal cues, but also the ability to connect and relate. This can be on a personal level or as an organizer of groups. In "Tipping Point," Malcolm Gladwell identifies *connectors* as people with a particular and rare set of social gifts" [11]. They know large numbers of people and are in the habit of making introductions. Their scope extends across an array of social, cultural, professional, and economic circles, and they make a habit of introducing people who work or live in different circles. They "link us up with the world…people with a special gift for bringing the world together". Those skilled in relationship management respond to others in a way that creates a connection, using both verbal and nonverbal modes of communication. In his book "Flourish," Seligman describes four ways to react to any situation: Active/Constructive, Passive/Constructive, Active/Destructive, and Passive/Destructive [12].

For example, on hearing of a colleague's raise and promotion, an active constructive response will show enthusiasm and interest, maintain eye contact, and ask questions to draw the teller in. A more passive response is to say, "Congratulations, you deserved it," with little or no emotion. Actively destructive responses will remind the teller of increased responsibility, time away from home and higher taxes. They will exhibit negative nonverbal communication in tone of voice or facial expression. The passively destructive person won't even acknowledge the news and may bring up an unrelated topic. How often in surgical training did we want to emulate the skilled clinician who could accurately and constructively help us improve? "After you set the needle at 45°, the anastomosis went more smoothly," as opposed to "I don't know how you got through sewing that with your left hand, but it's open…for now."

Nature Versus Nurture: The Biology of Emotion

More primitive organisms required near instantaneous responses to threats to survive. Further, basic regulation of physiologic function and movement was required. The brainstem and amygdala serve these functions, with the olfactory lobe as the main interaction with the surrounding environment. As our brains evolved, emotions developed before the recognition of emotions. Fight or flight was reflexive [13]. With the emergence of the limbic system came the ability to remember previous experiences and feel wider ranges of emotion. It remains our pleasure center. In psychopathology, the amygdala and limbic region have been implicated as a key neural region in emotional regulation.

With evolution and the specialized functions of the ever-enlarging neocortex, humans could now experience wide ranges of nuanced emotion. Concomitantly, neural pathways developed to modulate the primitive forebrain and the integrative amygdala. This region is essential to learning the emotional significance of cues in the environment. It is not static. The white matter of the frontal lobe grows through the end of adolescences and into early adulthood [14]. Liston and colleagues have shown that white matter tracts between prefrontal–basal ganglia and posterior fiber tracts continue to develop across childhood into adulthood, but only tracts between the prefrontal cortex and basal ganglia are correlated with impulse control. This may also explain why childhood reactions to impulses are so variable, since neural pathway development is incomplete [15]. In some individuals, these control pathways do not develop and taken to extreme, lead to sociopathic behavior.

The earliest studies on the brain and emotion centered on observed changes in personality after stroke, trauma, or surgical resection of these critical neural connections. More recently, functional magnetic resonance imaging (MRI) has given us even greater insight into where emotional intelligence may lie anatomically. It is now clear that the ability to recognize nonverbal cues (facial expression, tone of voice, word versus non-word sound) is complex and requires integration of disparate stimuli. Kreifelts examined functional MRI in a series of healthy adults who were presented with various words or non-word sounds, and human versus inanimate pictures [16]. In some cases, the words were spoken in either a happy or angry tone. Degree of activation in multiple areas of the brain was correlated with results from pre-study EQ testing. Subjects with higher EQ showed more activity in right posterior middle temporal gyrus during periods where integration of voice and facial expression was required. Of interest, in all subjects, the amygdala responded strongly to images of human faces but not voice. What remains to be seen is to what extent brain plasticity and learned responses to life events enhances these pathways [17].

Traumatic events of childhood clearly are correlated with later depression, yet not everyone with Early Life Stress (ELS) develops depression. Cisler mapped the emotion regulation network in a group of women who had ELS; some subsequently became clinical depressed while others had no such history [18]. Higher activity in the prefrontal cortex was seen in the resilient group, and more activation in the primitive amygdala in those with depression.

Surgeons deal with traumatic events daily. How they process these stimuli may be colored by early experiences and biology. Although one may feel doomed by biology, it is also clear that brain plasticity allows new neural pathways to form and mature throughout life. With an increasing recognition of burnout among physicians, comes the recognition that the antidote is not to reduce work hours, or hire scribes, but rather it is to reignite passion and perseverance into the workplace. Lee and Duckworth describe the stamina associated with high achievers as "grit." This is the attitude, forged by a love of what one is doing, that drives us to a goal despite sacrifices or easier paths. Grit compensates for middle of the road test scores or athletic ability. "Gritty" organizations align corporate mission and instill passion for the cause. They imbue a clear sense of purpose [19]. (You can calculate your own grittiness online at angeladuckworth.com/grit-scale.) It is ever more clear that the traits of optimism and resilience are key to success in surgery and joy in life.

Emotional Intelligence in Medical Practice and Leadership Roles

While having greater insight into one's feelings should correlate with success in leading others, supportive data in the medical field is not robust. Traditionally leaders in medicine have been selected on clinical or research accomplishments, not on their ability to manage themselves and mentor others. That said, one could easily argue that the need for such informed and consistent leadership has never been greater.

There is much information that would argue that physicians are experiencing considerable emotional stress due to a host of financial and other pressures that are dramatically changing both the practice of medicine and how doctors perceive their role in society. A survey of 1951 full-time physicians and scientists from four geographically separated medical schools noted that 20% had significant depressive symptoms [20]. Depression and anxiety scores were higher in young physicians (<35 years of age) than in their more senior colleagues. Relevant to this discussion, the very highest depression and anxiety levels were noted in surgeons; the lowest scores were recorded in emergency medicine physicians who had high acuity challenges but "controllable lifestyles." This suggests that the context in which the stress occurs (e.g. the degree of personalization, total work hours) has more to do with adverse emotional effects then the level of stress itself.

These differences are apparent in medical students and residents. Indeed, deficiencies may be exacerbated during training. Chew et al. administered the Mayer-Salovey-Caruso Emotional Intelligence Test (MSCEIT) to 163 first and final year medical students in Malaysia [21]. They correlated EQ with performance on standardized exams as well as clinical performance during rotations. There was a stronger correlation of higher EQ and performance in final year students than first year, reflecting the importance of resilience and humanism in successfully completing medical school. First year students, who were only age 18, were more focused on standardized knowledge testing. Many came into medical school with a degree of ambivalence toward a career in medicine as their own insight into emotional regulation (and neural pathways) were still developing. In a related study of American medical students, optimism, measured in the self-awareness realm, was correlated with higher satisfaction in course work and eventual National Board of Medical Examiners shelf examinations [22]. In a classic longitudinal study from UCSF, students with behavioral or emotional issues during medical school were much more likely to have subsequent malpractice cases or censure from medical boards [23].

In a study of nursing students, Beauvis correlated several realms of EQ, spirituality and resilience to academic success [24]. A similar pattern emerged to that of the Chew study. For younger undergraduate students, the only component of EQ that correlated to success was perceiving emotions, and that effect was moderate. In contrast, high performing graduate nursing students had overall higher total EQ with significant strength in facilitating thoughts and managing emotions. Finally, an overall strong association with academic success was seen with spirituality, however there may be selection bias as the nursing school studied was supported by a religious order.

Although surgeons are often accused of having poor social skills, in fact the opposite is true. Studies show they are strong in many realms. In a study by Stanton, 148 British psychiatrists and surgeons were assessed for EQ [25]; their overall scores were similar. Psychiatrists scored strongly in the subsets of empathy, self-awareness and impulse control. Surgeons had higher subscores in areas of self-regard, stress tolerance, and optimism. These traits inspire patient confidence, as no one wants to hear their surgeon say, "I hope I can help you…".

While it is obvious that an improved understanding of one's emotions is the ideal first step in this process, achieving personal insight is often difficult. In designing a recent study of 43 highly successful business leaders, Bennis and Thomas postulated that the "more modern" leader would have fundamentally different skills and tactics than CEO's of a more traditional era [26]. Yet, their subsequent research demonstrated that both sets of leaders were remarkably similar.

One common experience was particularly revealing. A majority of those interviewed described an unplanned and usually traumatic incident in mid-life which caused them to reformat their personal views of achievement and develop a higher level of empathy for others. In nearly every instance, they credited this specific response for their improved leadership performance.

Can I Improve My EQ?

The key constituents of emotional intelligence are self-assessment and empathy. Most workers in the field believe EI is not static but is a set of skills that can be learned with commitment and behavioral modeling [10, 27]. Those identified as true "servant" leaders have developed these skills, including conflict management, open communication, persuasiveness and change management. The ability to inspire through public speaking is coupled with drawing out other's opinions and building consensus.

Goleman [28] elucidated three key questions that you should ask yourself. Although they are in the context of increased EQ, they are a vital part of any self-reflection.

1. What are the differences between how you see yourself and how others see you?
2. What matters to you?
3. What changes will you make to achieve your goals?

Many of the skills seen in high EQ individuals are an inherent part of their personalities or learned during childhood and adolescence. Social norms are reinforced and the ability to read a group becomes increasingly important. Surgeons self-select because of personality traits that are rewarded throughout training and practice, many of which require some distancing oneself from emotion. Personal performances inside and outside the operating room are also measured and areas of opportunity for growth can be identified through comparison of one's own results with benchmarks and best practices. Such honest self-examination makes one open to learning from others even if it is often difficult to precisely quantitate our own strengths and weaknesses. Edward Deming, the father of process improvement, made it clear that you can't improve something that you don't measure.

Although there are multiple tools for EQ measurement [29], we have focused on three processes when assessing EQ in our medical staff leaders; the goal is to identify specific areas of strength and weakness and design plans to optimize performance. These are the Meyer-Salovey-Caruso Emotional Intelligence Test (MSCEIT); [9]; the Thomas-Kilmann Conflict mode analysis [30]; and the 360 evaluation. Taken together with appropriate interpretation and coaching, we have observed growth in our leaders' performance.

The MSCEIT analyzes specific tasks in each of the four areas of EI: self-awareness; self-management; social awareness; and relationship management. Test takers are assessed on their ability to identify emotions expressed by faces or pictures, appreciate the effects of mood on problem solving, and define how emotions are generated. Finally, the interaction of emotions in analyzing situations in ourselves and others is quantified by presentation of various scenarios. As in any test of this type, validation questions will reveal if the subject is attempting to present themselves in a favorable light. The eight specific sections are outlined In Table 5.1 (adapted from Mayer Caruso and Salovey [9]).

In our own assessment of emerging physician leaders at Cedars Sinai, we found strong self-management skills, with a wider variation in social awareness and relationship management. This is not surprising, given the selection bias of those who go into medicine, are trained to be self-reliant, and are taught to become objective

Table 5.1 Four basic abilities that are a component of Emotional Intelligence

Ability	Test sections	Question types
Identifying	Faces	Identify subtle emotions in faces
	Pictures	Identify emotions in complex landscapes and designs
Using	Facilitation	Knowledge of how moods impact thinking
	Sensations	Relate various feeling sensations to emotions
Understanding	Changes	Multiple choice questions about how emotions change over time
	Blends	Multiple choice emotion vocabulary definitions
Managing	Emotion management	Indicate effectiveness of various solutions to internal problems
	Emotional relations	Indicate effectiveness of various solutions to problems involving other people

Fig. 5.1 Styles of Conflict resolution (Copyright © 2009–2018 by Kilmann Diagnostics. All rights reserved. Original figure is available at: http://www. kilmanndiagnostics.com/ overview-thomas-kilmann-conflict-mode-instrument-tki)

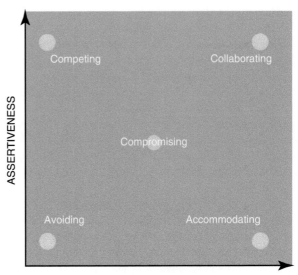

in the face of pain and suffering. This baseline helped us focus training in the important aspects of social skills in influencing group behaviors.

Although there are four realms to emotional intelligence, for leaders, success many times rests on their ability to resolve conflict. Conflict is not necessarily negative; opposing viewpoint may bring clarity to a situation. The Thomas Kilmann Conflict Mode Instrument (TKI) was an outgrowth of work in the 1960's on managerial styles [30]. It recognizes that there are gradations of assertiveness and cooperativeness in any conflict negotiation. Assertiveness is the degree to which you try to satisfy your own needs, cooperativeness in the degree to which you try to satisfy others needs and be receptive to their ideas. These are not mutually exclusive. Depending on the situation, each style may be appropriate.

If one places assertiveness on the Y axis and cooperativeness on the X axis, five styles become apparent (Fig. 5.1):

- Being both unassertive and uncooperative is consistent with an **avoiding** style. This may be appropriate in conflicts with low impact that are in the process of resolving themselves, or for which you may need to buy time to become more prepared. The risks include declining workplace relationships as people become uncomfortable working through differences.
- Those who **accommodate** are high in cooperativeness, but low in assertiveness. You are willing to concede your own needs for the good of others. This can support others and smooth ruffled feathers, but if done excessively, causes loss of self-respect and motivation.
- Being highly assertive and uncooperative can lead to rapid victories and protection of self-interest. This **competitive** style forces active debate of one's own

position and the need to justify it. Appropriate in highly time constrained nego-tiations, it can also lead to escalation and deadlock as well as poor decisions and resentment by the loser.

- **Compromising** styles try to find middle ground. Both parties give up something as well as retain key components that are of value to them. Compromise main-tains relationships and fairness, but the solution is often suboptimal. Expediency is the tradeoff for highest quality.
- The most time-consuming negation style is **collaboration.** Parties strive for a "win win." Through a structure of understanding that both likely share many common values and goals, early agreement is sought. With openness and trust, the areas of disagreement are dissected and both parties challenged to create innovative solutions that are better than each's initial proposal. Done well, col-laborative negotiations increase team cohesiveness and mutual respect. If not facilitated tactfully, exposed vulnerabilities may lead to exploitation and hurt feelings around sensitive issues.

We were somewhat surprised to find that our leadership group primarily dealt with conflict by accommodation rather than avoidance and compromise. Only one physician scored strongly in collaboration; this was a member of the voluntary med-ical staff who has been successful in organizing community-based practitioners. We were encouraged that, when the group as a whole was retested after a year, we saw a shift in avoidance behavior with increases in compromise and collaboration. Many organizations offer negotiation training for leaders emphasizing that conflict is not only unavoidable but, channeled properly, can lead to innovation and increased performance.

Perhaps one of the greatest innovative disruptions in performance management is 360° feedback. Gone are days when subordinates were evaluated only by their supervisors, who themselves were responsible to a level higher in the organizational chart. Personal success was narrowly defined, and corporate cultures focused on shareholder value, or for academic medical centers, on grants, patient care dollars and charitable giving. A true understanding of mission, vision and core values was lacking. Personal growth and the ability to manage and supervise to the mission required a far greater understanding of one's own style, strengths, and areas of opportunity. The 360 also requires high levels of trust and self-awareness to yield meaningful behavioral change. Selection of the feedback tool, the raters, the method of feedback and the integration into the culture are key decision points to be consid-ered. In general, the more feedback from multiple sources, the better [31]. The abil-ity to lead teams that are multigenerational and multidisciplinary is an increasingly important skill, different from the leadership learned in the operating room.

At Cedars Sinai, 360 evaluations are available on an individual basis, and chairs receive pooled feedback from their faculty, including trends and comparison to other departments. Other organizations incorporate 360° evaluations into the culture beginning with onboarding. There is an explicit expectation to receive and give feedback at all levels. Done well, 360° evaluations not only enhance personal per-formance, but also can guide an organization to develop programs in areas consistently identified as high impact. The risks of the 360 is to focus on deficiencies and then not have the resources in place to optimize individuals' performance. It is vital to tie the evaluations of the individual to clear understanding of the organization's goals. If the mission is the service of the local urban community, cultural awareness should be included; if it is to compete in a highly specialized technology transfer environment, the ability to understand big data and communicate that clearly is paramount.

As with any form of evaluation, standardized testing is but one component of an overall program of personal and professional development. You can be coached, read self-help books, and do exercises to better read facial expressions. But the journey as a leader, and in finding joy in one's life, comes from within. Souba describes the "Inward Journey of Leadership" as a continuous process of self-reflection, discovery and growth [32]. It focuses on accurate self-awareness, not defined by the size of one's CV. It is expanded by seeking feedback and constantly comparing your interactions with others to your inner values. It is genuine human connections, forged through both adversity and success, that is the greatest tool in understanding our own emotions and how we are perceived.

These insights have been useful in assisting the "difficult" physician who disparages and turns over associates repeatedly. These poor working relationships were rarely the result of the skill level of the new colleague. Far more often they reflected some other issue entirely, such as the senior surgeon's discontent over perceived status in the organization. While it was rarely easy to initiate, a frank discussion which identified the key driver and addressed it has been a far more efficient tact then recycling yet another young physician into an adverse environment. In addition to exploring the obvious (i.e. what the senior physician could do to improve the comfort and performance level of his juniors,) the difficult conversation of other external factors comes into play. Done sensitively, deeper personal insight was gained. Quite often, this self-knowledge translated to more collegial behavior in other areas.

Such successful "teaching" of emotional intelligence requires an immediate and real-life context to both stimulate and reward skill acquisition. Personal insight is an important element, but it is useful to remember that efforts are most effective when directed toward modification of *behavior* not *personality*. The goal is a practical one—minimization of poor personal interactions by recognition and self-correction of non-productive behavior. While motivated learners can occasionally gain these skills by self-study, the presence of role models and mentors can greatly facilitate the process. Surgical leaders must always be aware that their personal conduct and equanimity sends a strong signal to the entire group.

How Can I Improve My Own EQ?

Although imbedded patterns of behavior and interactions may be hard to break, there is evidence that insight and some specific exercises can develop EQ skills [22]. Since self-awareness requires the ability to recognize one's emotional state and how perceptions are altered, some form of introspection is key Journaling creates a dedicated time to review the day and reflect on emotions felt and triggers that were recognized. In addition to looking within, asking for feedback from trusted friends and colleagues can help frame your actions and feelings within a broader and more objective context. As you become more aware of your physiologic response to stress, you will be able to "slow down and think" before your primitive brainstem takes over. Self-management feeds on this recognition of impulsivity and the ability to put a temporary hard stop on a proposed action.

There is a revealing story of a superb senior airline pilot who was in the simulator. Multiple emergencies were being created for him. As things began to accelerate, he took off his watch and spent a few seconds winding it (this was years ago) then sorted things out. During the debriefing he was asked about the watch. "I never grabbed the wrong lever or crashed the plane while I was winding my watch," he replied. These individuals exhibit extreme equanimity in the face of chaos ("Zen Masters"). We all recognize them - seek their counsel. Consider yoga or meditation to become more aware of your body and mind. Take responsibility when thing go wrong, and look objectively at the decisions made, and different paths that could be taken.

Social awareness cannot occur if you are in your own head rather than the situation at hand. You will fail to appreciate body language or anticipate what the other person is saying. Premature and often inaccurate conclusions predictably follow. The key is to listen and assess, sometimes a difficult feat for a surgeon who daily moves forward proactively with limited information. Perhaps the greatest skill is to put yourself in the other person's position. We have found this useful when counseling other physicians while in our leadership roles. Sometimes a simple, "what would you do, if you were sitting in my chair?" brings clarity.

Relationship management coalesces the other three skills. Being available to those you lead and setting a strong example of drawing in diverse opinions sets a tone of collaboration and respect. It is important to acknowledge and praise those who have contributed to a goal and take personal responsibility when there are missteps of those you lead. It involves humor and strength…and hoping for luck and good timing.

Conclusion

Our emotional intelligence has a chance to grow if we let ourselves be aware and be present every day. We can see it in the body language of surgeons who were residents together, when they are recounting their internship days over a beer at a national meeting; we experience the sense of flow during a presentation when we are connecting with our audience, or we relish it in a spontaneous sharing of advice with our teenage daughter over a coffee at Starbucks. And perhaps we feel it most poignantly, when we watch a friend, colleague, or mentor self-destruct a long and brilliant career, because of their lack of self-awareness and self-control.

In the highly demanding environment of modern medical practice, positive interpersonal interactions are necessary to optimize clinical and academic productivity. Searching for a better understanding of others has the additional value of enhancing insights into our own actions and reactions, and improving personal satisfaction [33, 34]. As the value of emotional intelligence becomes even more evident, it is quite likely that more formal assessments of these skills will be used in selecting and training the surgical leaders of tomorrow.

References

1. Boyatzis RE. The competent manager: a model for effective performance. New York: Wiley; 1982.
2. Spencer L, Spencer S. Competence at work. New York: Wiley; 1993.
3. Goleman D. What makes a leader? Harv Bus Rev. 1998;76(6):93–102.
4. Clavien PA, Deiss J. Ten tips for choosing an academic chair. Nature. 2015;519:286–7.
5. Beydler KW. The role of emotional intelligence in perioperative nursing and leadership. AORN. 2017;106:317–23.
6. Wang L, Tao H, Bowers BJ, et al. When nurse emotional intelligence matters: how transformational leadership influences intent to stay. J Nurs Manag. 2018;26:358–65.
7. Mintz LJ, Stoller JK. A systematic review of physician leadership and emotional intelligence. J Grad Med Educ. 2014;6:21–31.
8. Goleman D. Emotional intelligence. New York: Bantam Books; 1995.
9. Mayer JD, Caruso D, Salovey P. Emotional intelligence meets traditional standards for intelligence. Intelligence. 2000;27:267–98.
10. Taylor GJ, Parker JD, Bagby RM. Emotional intelligence and the emotional brain: points of convergence and implications for psychoanalysis. J Am Acad Psychoanal. 1999;27:339–54.
11. Gladwell M. The tipping point: how little things can make a big difference. New York: Little Brown and Company; 2002.
12. Seligman M. Flourish: a visionary new understanding of happiness and well- being. New York: Simon and Schuster; 2011.
13. Maren S, Quirk GJ. Neuronal signaling of fear memory. Nat Rev Neurosci. 2004;5:844–52.
14. Lenroot RK, Giedd JN. Brain development in children and adolescents: insights from anatomical magnetic resonance imaging. Neurosci Biobehav Rev. 2006;30:718–29.
15. Liston C, Watts R, Tottenham N, et al. Frontostriatal microstructure modulates efficient recruitment of cognitive control. Cereb Cortex. 2006;16:553–60.
16. Kreifelts B, Ethofer T, Huberle E, Grodd W, Wildgruber D. Association of trait emotional intelligence and individual fMRI-activation patterns during the perception of social signals from voice and face. Hum Brain Mapp. 2010;31:979–91.
17. Schwartz JM, Begley S. The mind and the brain: neuroplasticity and the power of mental force. New York: Regan Books/Harper Collins Publishers; 2002.
18. Cisler JM, James GA, Tripath S, et al. Differential functional connectivity within and emotion regulation neural network among individuals resilient and susceptible to the depressogenic effects of early life stress. Psychol Med. 2013;43:507–18.
19. Lee TH, Duckworth AL. Organizational grit: turning passion and perseverance into performance. HBR, Sept–Oct 2018. p. 98–105.
20. Schindler BA, Novack DH, Cohen DG, et al. The impact of the changing health care environment on the health and well-being of faculty at four medical schools. Acad Med. 2006;81:27–34.
21. Chew BH, Zain AM, Hassan F. Emotional intelligence and academic performance in first and final year medical students: a cross-sectional study. BMC Med Educ. 2013;13:44–50.
22. Artino AR, LaRochelle JS, Durning SJ. Second year medical students' motivational beliefs, emotions, and achievement. Med Educ. 2010;13:1203–12.

23. Papadakis MA, Teherani A, Banach MA, et al. Disciplinary action by-medical boards and prior behavior in medical school. NEJM. 2005;353:2673–82.
24. Beauvais AM, Stewart JG, Denisco S, Beauvais JE. Factors related to academic success among nursing students: a descriptive correlational research study. Nurs Educ Today. https://doi.org/10.1016/j.nedt.2013.12.005.
25. Stanton C, Sethi FN, Dale O, et al. Comparison of emotional intelligence between psychiatrists and surgeons. Psychiatrist. 2011;35:125–9.
26. Bennis WG, Thomas RJ. Crucibles of leadership. Harv Bus Rev. 2002;80:39–45.
27. Bradberry T, Greaves J. Emotional Intelligence 2.0. San Diego: Talent Smart Press; 2009.
28. Goleman D, Nevarez M. https://hbr.org/2018/08/boost-your-emotional-intelligence-with-these-3-questions. 16 Aug 2018.
29. Boyatzis RE. The behavioral level of emotional intelligence and its measurement. Front Psych. 2018;9:1439–43.
30. Thomas KW, Kilmann RH. Thomas-Kilmann conflict mode instrument. Mountain View, CA: Xicom, a subsidiary of CPP, Inc.; 1974.
31. Peiperl MA. Getting 360 degree feedback right. Harv Bus Rev. 2001;79:142–7.
32. Souba WW. The inward journey of leadership. J Surg Res. 2006;131:159–67.
33. Taylor P, Funk C, Craighill P. Are we happy yet? Washington, DC: Pew Research Center; 2006.
34. Csikszentmihalyi M. Flow: the psychology of optimal experience. New York: Harper & Row; 1990.

Practical Tips for Developing Leadership Skills Early in a Career

6

Sarah Tevis, Herbert Chen, and Gregory Kennedy

Introduction

When we think of leaders in surgery, Division Chiefs, Chairs of Surgery, and Presidents of national organizations come to mind. However, surgeons can be leaders the day they start their first job. After finishing training, new faculty are often focused on the day to day tasks of getting settled into their new institution and role. This is precisely when surgeons should establish themselves as a leader and build leadership skills. This will allow new faculty to achieve their short and long term goals and grow to ultimately be known as a leader in their field. Effective leaders inspire others to want to build a productive and successful team and improve performance. This is true for the team of nurses, MAs, and schedulers in clinic, the members of a research program or lab, the multi-disciplinary team in the operating room, and the team of residents and medical students caring for patients. Good leaders find that the people they work with every day go out of their way to help them reach their goals and see that the daily pressures of starting a new job and building a practice are eased with a well-functioning team. Unfortunately, many faculty struggle to establish themselves as a leader as they embark on their first job. In this chapter, we hope to outline the leadership skills it takes to be effective in these first few years and how attaining these skills early on will translate into a successful leadership style that will serve a young surgeon throughout their career (Table 6.1).

S. Tevis
Department of Surgery, University of Colorado, Denver, CO, USA
e-mail: sarah.tevis@ucdenver.edu

H. Chen · G. Kennedy (✉)
Department of Surgery, University of Alabama at Birmingham,
Birmingham, AL, USA
e-mail: hchen@uabmc.edu; gkennedy@uabmc.edu

© Springer Nature Switzerland AG 2019
M. R. Kibbe, H. Chen (eds.), *Leadership in Surgery*, Success in Academic
Surgery, https://doi.org/10.1007/978-3-030-19854-1_6

Table 6.1 Leadership skills: an outline of the skills for junior faculty to be effective and translate skills into a leadership style that will serve them throughout their career

	Leadership principle	Short summary
1	Have a Clear Vision	Write a purpose statement, set goals, and revisit your goals to ensure you are staying on track
2	Seek Out Opportunities	Look for opportunities in everyday tasks, fully engage, and maximize your participation
3	Optimize Efficiency	Use each minute of the day to accomplish the tasks that serve your long-term purpose
4	Be Positive	Assume good intentions in others, see the opportunity in challenges
5	Engage the Team	Provide a clear vision, encourage your team, and give them the tools and support to succeed
6	Develop a Sense of Identity	Create a team environment, provide positive and negative feedback
7	Be Selfless	Be the first to volunteer for tasks, show that you are willing to pitch in and help out
8	Get Involved	Join societies, volunteer for and be active on committees
9	Ask for Help	Ask mentors for advice, delegate and follow up on tasks

Have a Clear Vision

Good leaders have self-awareness, discipline, and are able to manage themselves. In order to achieve their goals, leaders must have a clear vision for the future, be able to communicate that vision to others, and generate enthusiasm around the importance of the work. Excellent leaders develop their vision around their passion and, with the end in mind, are able to focus and work toward achieving their goals. When leaders have a clear vision, team members identify common goals and values and will align with the overall vision. This leads to consensus building, teamwork, and cohesiveness as the team works together to accomplish tasks in line with the shared vision.

Developing a list of short term goals in 1, 3, and 5 year increments can ensure leaders are productive and constantly building toward their long term goals. Early career surgeons have many areas of focus including clinical, research, educational, and administrative. Therefore, it is important to develop goals, as well as a timeline with appropriate milestones, in each area. It is also important to prioritize goals and place an emphasis on achieving early wins in high priority areas. Posting these goals and timelines in a visible place, such as on a desk or as a calendar reminder, can serve as a periodic reminder and help leaders stay on schedule. Scheduling mentor meetings monthly or quarterly can also serve as a time to assess if milestones are being met and either celebrate successes or re-evaluate project plans and goals.

By staying organized and setting specific goals, a clear purpose will be pervasive in all activities taken on by the team and team members will be able to work together toward a common vision. Beginning with an end in mind will ensure success in staying focused and reaching both short and long term goals [1]. A productive, rewarding career can be developed by working hard with self-management, tackling short term attainable goals, and building a high performing, cohesive team.

Seek Out Opportunities

Junior faculty are often asked to serve on multiple departmental or institutional committees. It is important to evaluate the opportunities for committee involvement and align committee service with overall goals. For example, for a surgeon who is interested in becoming a residency program director or who specializes in educational research, serving on the Graduate Medical Education trainee curriculum committee would be worthwhile and may dovetail nicely with ongoing research projects. Similarly, getting involved with societal committees as junior faculty can facilitate networking, leadership positions within the committees, and may serve as a way to rise to leadership positions within the society.

The caveat to committee involvement is that simply being a committee member is insufficient. In order to ascend to leadership positions, a positive attitude, strong work ethic, and meaningful contributions to the committee's work are necessary. This may involve volunteering to take the lead on a manuscript the committee is writing, serving as a recorder and point of contact for the committee, or organizing an event for the committee at a national conference. Framing these seemingly mundane tasks as opportunities and facing them with enthusiasm demonstrates the generosity, hard work, and dedication of a leader [2]. Furthermore, these behaviors will be noticed by leaders in the field, will ensure early career successes, and will lead to promotion to leadership roles.

Optimize Efficiency

William Penn is quoted as saying, "Time is what we want most, but what we use worst." Efficient use of time allows surgeons to accomplish each day's work, which thereby allows for achievement of long term goals and maintenance of work life balance. Time management skills involve the ability to plan and prioritize, delegate, and scheduling each week to ensure protected time for research and writing. There are many mundane tasks including emails, phone calls, charting, and administrative tasks that can fill up days at a time if not managed. Keeping a list of tasks on hand for when the operating room is running late, a meeting is unexpectedly cancelled, or while waiting for a patient to emerge from anesthesia in the operating room can facilitate utilizing these 30–60 min windows of time to complete these tasks before they pile up. The ability to complete these tasks quickly and on time may allow for the much needed time to write an abstract, prepare a talk, or attend a child's soccer game or school play.

It is also important to have a weekly schedule to separate clinical, research, and personal time. Figure 6.1 demonstrates an example schedule where clinical time is grouped to maximize efficiency and time for research and writing is specifically laid out. In addition to keeping a personal schedule, it is important to communicate this schedule to any administrative assistants or surgery schedulers who have the ability to add events to the calendar. For example, utilizing a color coding system to demarcate these broad scheduling categories as well as to note within categories when it is acceptable to add appointments. For instance, during blocks of time dedicated to research, it may not be possible for schedulers to add any surgeries, meetings, or

Time	Monday	Tuesday	Wednesday	Thursday	Friday	Saturday	Sunday
6	Write	Write	Conferences	Write	Dictate	Write	Write
7							
8				Add On	Elective		
9				Cases	Outpatient		
10					Cases		
11							
12	Research	Research	Elective				
1			Cases		Inpatient		
2				Clinic	Cases	Family Time	Family Time
3							
4							
5							
6							
7							
8	Family Time	Family Time	Family Time	Family Time	Family Time		
9							
10							

Fig. 6.1 A typical week from GK's calendar his first year on surgical faculty in 2007

appointments on Monday so that time may be spent in the lab or writing manuscripts. While schedulers would have the ability to add research meetings on Tuesday mornings and any surgeries added outside of the clinical time frames would require direct communication for approval to schedule. It can also be beneficial to meet with administrative assistants on a weekly basis to review the schedule for the upcoming week. This will guarantee that the schedule remains controlled and ensure protected time to complete the tasks needed to meet short and long term goals.

In addition to scheduling work related activities, it is also important to schedule personal activities and include them on a work calendar. This allows an administrative assistant or surgery scheduler to avoid scheduling clinical or administrative tasks during important personal events. The phrase "work life balance" is being abandoned for the more reasonable "work life integration" in an era where surgeons juggle clinical responsibilities, research, administrative duties, family, community involvement, and self-care. To safeguard against burnout and maintain wellness, it is important to schedule time for exercise, relaxation, and quality time with family and friends. This may require creative scheduling based on individual preference and self-reflection about what time of day is personally most productive. For example, if there is a half day program at a child's school, it may require working after bedtime or early in the morning to complete the tasks for that day or if there is an hour gap every Tuesday it may be a good time to go to the gym during the day. Regardless, when important personal or family events arise, it is important to put these events on the calendar with the same priority as other scheduled work events.

Be Positive

The downfall of many young academic surgeons is negativity. An overly negative perspective can change how every task is viewed and in the long-term can affect productivity. Furthermore, negativity can influence interactions with colleagues and superiors. By maintaining positivity and demonstrating enthusiasm, the likelihood that superiors will provide local opportunities to shine, speak positively about young staff, and recommend staff for national committees and organizations. The opportunist approach ultimately gives rise to leadership opportunities as a young surgeon's potential is realized at their institution and nationally. Individuals who approach obligations as opportunities for growth and success are more likely to be perceived as a role model to others in surgical department, and this does not go unrecognized by the senior leaders [2].

In addition to leading to more opportunities, maintaining a positive outlook will allow colleagues and team members to see a junior faculty as someone they want to follow. A positive person is typically someone who can generate energy and engage others. Attracting a diverse group of the best candidates and engaging them in research or clinical work will allow a leader to efficiently and effectively advance an agenda. It is much easier to attract the top colleagues, residents, and medical students as a positive collaborator who others want to work with.

Engage the Team

Engagement of the team is a critical skill that is necessary to develop as leadership positions are obtained. A team that is engaged with the leader's vision is much more likely to work effectively towards the goals of the team. How does one go about engaging a team? This can be a challenging task but can be broken down into four simple steps:

1. First, the clear vision that was discussed earlier needs to be effectively communicated to the team so every member understands the vision and purpose of the team. Without this clarity, the team will lose sight of the goal, potentially become distracted by unrelated issues, and will ultimately fail. Conversely, when team members see the importance of what they are doing, they will work better together and will work tirelessly to achieve the goals. Frequent team meetings where the importance of the work and the short and long term goals are emphasized can ensure all team members are on the same page and working toward the same vision.
2. Encourage the team's hard work and accomplishments. As they work hard to achieve the standards and goals that have been set, team members will continue to do their best work if they are encouraged along the way. This can be as simple as saying "thank you!" or "great work!" or a larger expression of gratitude, such as a team dinner or outing. Influential leaders are champions and cheerleaders for their team.
3. Set new challenges. Challenging existing processes along the way can be a key factor in successful innovation. Many projects fail because of adherence to the status quo. Constant reevaluation of the team's processes and acceptance of input from team members about how things might be improved can stimulate the team to improve and be creative in the process. Team to improve and be creative with the process.

4. Provide a collaborative environment. Mistakes will happen and how a team addresses those mistakes determines if the team fails or is successful. Approaching issues as opportunities leads to collaboration and a shared team struggle to overcome challenges. All team members must feel empowered to raise concerns so that the team can grow and work effectively. Team morale improves and new, creative ideas emerge when unique perspectives are encouraged and supported. This collaborative environment develops out of the team identity built by the leader.

Ultimately, the team is going to be much more engaged if they believe in the success of the project, they have a strong leader who can collaborate and build consensus, and they have a positive working environment. Effective team engagement is a priceless resource when building a career.

Develop a Sense of Identity

It is important for young leaders to develop a sense of team identity early on. Initially this may mean inviting the surgical team and their families to dinner or creating a logo for a skull cap and purchasing one for all team members (Fig. 6.2). These activities allow team members to get to know the leader and each other, creates a sense of camaraderie, and develops trust and loyalty amongst the team. As trust and loyalty develop, these relationships will carry the team through all the ups and downs of managing a successful practice or implementing a successful research program and will establish a young faculty as a dependable leader.

In addition to the team environment, effective mentorship includes providing direct feedback to team members. This is a vitally important skill that requires work to

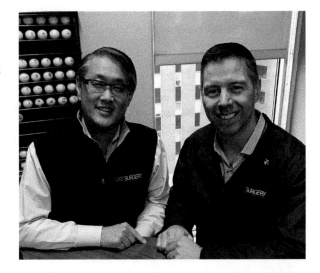

Fig. 6.2 GK and HC sporting their team branded jackets. These jackets are worn around the hospital, around town, and at national meetings. Such branding creates a sense of identity and camaraderie developing trust and loyalty between team members. All new faculty members are given a jacket when they arrive and are encouraged to wear it

develop in the early career years. Providing helpful critiques of a person's performance requires an understanding of what each job entails, a desire to create successful team members, and expectations that each team member will be accountable for their tasks. The term "providing feedback" frequently has negative connotations, but this is not just about correcting negative behaviors. Positive feedback is just as valuable because it encourages an individual to work hard, to continue exhibiting valued traits, and allows them to see the leader as a resource for their job performance and success. Strong leaders are willing to provide effective feedback and when leaders demonstrate the ability to provide feedback, even more leadership opportunities arise.

Defining an identity that is in line with career goals will help junior faculty come to mind when colleagues hear of opportunities. This leads to junior faculty having sponsors who actively advocate for their career development as opposed to more passive mentors who offer advice to mentees. For example, sponsors may refer patients if a junior partner is trying to increase volume, share new community outreach activities, or suggest the junior faculty for a committee, leadership position, or speaking engagement.

Be Selfless

Leadership takes time, effort, energy, and hard work. A good leader is one who is not afraid to jump in and work. Leaders must be willing to make sacrifices to build trust and be engaged with the team. It is important to lead by example, especially when the team is tackling something particularly onerous. This may mean taking more call, teaching more medical student lectures, helping with data collection, etc. The bottom line is that colleagues are not going to follow someone who they don't feel works as hard as they do. This also means being willing to say, "Yes." Much too often a young faculty member is too busy worrying about her own progress and forgets that she is part of a larger community. After saying "No" a few times, opportunities will no longer be offered. A large part of being a leader is being willing to make sacrifices when needed to build trust and a sense of accomplishment, which allows the team to grow closer.

Get Involved

There are many regional and national surgical societies that a young surgeon can join. It is easy to become overwhelmed by choice, join too many organizations, or never really find a home in an organization. Joining an organization provides networking opportunities, committee and leadership involvement, and the opportunity to rise the ranks to leadership positions. When joining national organizations, it is important to have a strategy for potential roles in the organization and goals for participating in the organization. Joining an organization with aspirations to lead whether it be at the committee or organizational level, increase the likelihood of success in being an active member of the organization.

The first society many early career surgeons join is the "home society". This is usually a specialty organization—AAES for an endocrine surgeon, ASCRS for a colon and rectal surgeon, ASBrS for a breast surgeon, etc. A good early career goal is to submit abstracts to this society and attend this meeting yearly. In addition, it is a great idea to try to get involved in the home society early perhaps by volunteering for committee membership and following through by actively engaging in those committees. Before volunteering for a committee, consider what each committee does and how personal strengths and interests can align well with a committee. For example, joining the website committee would be a poor choice for someone who does not enjoy using technology and social media. Colleagues across the country comprise these committees and all successes and failures will be noticed.

In addition to a home society, there are many other non-specialty societies. These might include the American College of Surgeons, the Association of Academic Surgery, Society of University Surgeons, Society for Surgery of the Alimentary Tract, and other general academic societies. The reason to consider joining these types of organizations is to broaden a friendship and networking base and to gain more learning opportunities. Many of these organizations provide opportunities to lead committees early on and these are invaluable experiences as they will provide mentorship as well as knowledge. These organizations also have resources for career advancement including courses on career development, grant writing, leadership, etc. Finally, for research mentors, these non-specialty organizations are often more friendly to trainees and provide a forum for residents and students to present their work, which is important for junior faculty with mentees.

Ask for Help

Every good leader has many mentors he or she can point to over the years who have helped them achieve their goals. Asking these mentors for advice is a critical piece to improving leadership skills. Mentors can be helpful at every career stage and can be invaluable in developing leadership experience. In fact, the only mistake one can make is failing to ask for help when it is needed.

In addition to asking mentors for advice along the way, it is important to engage the entire team by trusting them to take on aspects of the team's work. Delegation allows team members to take ownership of the project and by giving up control it allows a diversity of ideas to enhance the success of the team's work. However, when delegating, it is important to follow up with team members to track progress and provide input. The team needs to know they can count on their leader and that their leader is available. Effective delegation provides stability for the team and can lead to improved productivity.

Summary

We hope that the principles outlined above will guide early career academic surgeons to build leadership skills. Strong leadership of others depends upon the ability to effectively lead oneself. By recognizing a clear vision and long term goals early in a career, being willing to develop skills and improve weaknesses, and being able to effectively engage colleagues and team members long term successes will be realized. It is essential to take advantage of early opportunities as hard work is quickly recognized by others. Early successes will lead to significant leadership opportunities for a dedicated, productive junior faculty member who can effectively organize and lead a team.

References

1. Covey SR. The 7 habits of highly effective people: restoring the character ethic. rev. ed. New York: Free Press; 2004.
2. Sanborn M. You don't need a title to be a leader: how anyone, anywhere, can make a positive difference. 1st WaterBrook Press ed. Colorado Springs, CO: WaterBrook Press; 2006.

Common Mistakes in Leadership

7

Jonathan D. Gates and David W. McFadden

Introduction

For the first edition of this monograph I was quite flattered when asked to contribute to a textbook on surgical leadership, until I was told I was invited to write the chapter about leadership mistakes. After an initial hesitation and false sense of insult, I decided "yes!" because over my past two decades of leadership in academic surgery I have unquestionably made a great deal of mistakes. Mistakes are valuable because you can only learn from them, and if shared, others may learn from them too. If you are not making mistakes, you are not trying hard enough. I decided, with the use of a few important references, to provide what I believe are the top mistakes that a surgical leader, or perhaps any leader, may make. I assure you that I have made them all, and unfortunately, I will unquestionably commit at least a few more during the remainder of my career. I ask the readers to review the reference list of classic articles and textbooks that are worthy of their study if they aspire to successful surgical leadership careers. For this second edition, I have asked my colleague and co-author, a newly minted Professor and Chairman, to add his perspective and expertise.

First, leadership matters! In Joseph Simone's words:" What makes great leaders is not a secret-they not only have grace under pressure, which means both courage and character, they remain focused on the important aspects of an issue in the midst of chaos, and they repeatedly articulate a consistent, simple public vision." It is also important to differentiate between leadership and management. It is often said that management means doing things right, whereas leadership is doing the right thing,

J. D. Gates
Department of Surgery, Hartford Hospital, University of Connecticut, Farmington, CT, USA
e-mail: Jonathan.gates@hhchealth.org

D. W. McFadden (✉)
Department of Surgery, University of Connecticut, Farmington, CT, USA
e-mail: dmcfadden@uchc.edu

© Springer Nature Switzerland AG 2019
M. R. Kibbe, H. Chen (eds.), *Leadership in Surgery*, Success in Academic Surgery, https://doi.org/10.1007/978-3-030-19854-1_7

and much more difficult. As a surgical leader you will need to be both a manager and a leader. Management issues tend to be urgent, the daily putting out of fires. They can be briefly satisfying in solving, but can and will get in the way of leadership issues, which are more important and often less immediately gratifying.

Peter F. Drucker was the most famous, prolific, and profound management thinker that ever lived. I recommend many of his works and will include them in my reference list. Many of his axioms can be applied to leadership.

The first and most important step in building leadership skills is to be self-aware of your own weaknesses and strengths, and to work on minimizing and improving them, respectively. Do not be afraid to seek counsel or coaching. Pursue feedback rather than waiting for it to happen. Ask yourself, when interviewing for a job, if your direct supervisor (Dean, Chair, CEO) is a mentoring individual. Often Chairs are hired without any support or promise for their own professional development. Perhaps there are a few natural leaders out there who do not need it, but not us. We have dozens of leadership and business school textbooks on our shelves, all of them read and highlighted. There are several more in our Amazon queues. None, however, has taught us as much as the one-on-one sessions we have had with the great mentors of our careers. Leadership, like surgery, is a lifelong learning experience. Embrace it. Both authors approached middle age by entering MBA programs.

In Halverson's article it is wisely stated that leadership is two sides of the same coin: self-management and team management. Self-management is based on emotional intelligence, which is the ability to manage oneself and one's relationships. We encourage you to read or review Daniel Goleman's salient works about emotional intelligence. Briefly, emotional intelligence comprises four essential domains: Self-awareness, self-management, social awareness, and social skills. This topic is elaborated upon in another chapter of this book. Goleman further divides leadership styles into authoritative, coaching, affiliative, democratic, pacesetting, and commanding. Bing Rikkers, in his wonderful Presidential Address to the Central Surgical Association, comments that surgical leaders must be able to use multiple leadership styles depending on the situation. He likens these to the golf clubs in one's bag that one appropriately deploys depending on the shot required. For example in the operating room, when there is a sudden injury to the right hepatic vein, a surgical leader would use a commanding leadership style, as using the democratic style or coaching style could be lethal. We continue to see many surgical leaders use the commanding, or "surgical mentality" style by default, in situations where affiliative or democratic leadership is far more appropriate.

Another important reference that we recommend to all serious readers and students of leadership is *Rules* by Donald Rumsfeld. Irrespective of whether you like his political beliefs and career, there are many pithy and profound rules that apply to business, government, military, and surgery. Many of them will be used in this chapter. So in the essence of brevity we would like to give you our Top 13 errors list. We apologize in advance for the curmudgeonly and frequent use of quotations. The 13 errors are not ranked in order of ignominy or priority, yet they also all interrelate at some level.

Number One: Failure to Appreciate that Institutions Do Not Love You Back

This is the first rule from Joseph V. Simone's classic and "a must read" manuscript entitled "Understanding Academic Medical Centers: Simone's Maxims ". Although at first blush this may sound cynical, one simply cannot presume the same respect or appreciation from an enterprise that one would from a friend or family member. You will be astonished that even the most wizened senior faculty believes that they somehow merit special dispensation because of their longevity, or past productivity, or sworn allegiance to an organization. Repeat after us: "What have you done for me, lately?" Simone refers to a colleague who opines that the only true job security is the ability to move to another position, because of professional independence. In these days of rotating Chief Executive Officers and Deans, it is sad to say that institutional loyalty to an individual, especially a chair, cannot be counted upon. Institutional lifespans are long, ours is ephemeral in comparison.

Although we will discuss this later, the concept of "tickets, or chits" should be mentioned here. Jerry Shuck, in his presidential address to the Central Surgical Association, presented the hypothesis that an individual is given a certain and fixed number of tickets when granted a leadership position. The number of tickets granted is a carefully guarded secret that this individual never knows until the last one is spent. The purpose of this digression is that when there is a change in leadership at the Dean or CEO level, the chair's reserve of tickets may precipitously decrease or disappear.

Number Two: Failure to Appreciate that Not Everyone in the Room Is as Interested in Team Success

Transitions are the riskiest time for the new leader, yet potentially can yield the greatest rewards. Much is written about the first 90 days of any transition and the need to learn about the culture of the new organization, as well as the need for transparency, clarity and repetitive delivery of the new message. There is much emphasis on the early definitive wins and the identification of allies who will help you carry that message forward. Remember: culture is the most fundamental framework of teamwork and reflects the heart and soul of the team. Culture can be good or bad. Do not underestimate the power of the pre-existing culture for it has persisted for a reason. Do not assume it is for the good of the team. As Peter Drucker was fond of saying "Culture eats strategy for breakfast."

Yes, we are surgeons who thrive on the art and science of medicine and would do anything for a colleague, patient or family in need. But, do not always assume that everyone on that new team shares your most fundamental values, good will, and resolute understanding of the power of teamwork. Failure to realize that you cannot convince some that change is needed will continue to plague the most fundamental improvements.

Some members of the team will never admit that change is needed nor have an alternate plan for the organization. These individuals may spread anarchy for the sake of anarchy. This is often surreptitiously performed through a carefully crafted pre-existing subcultural labyrinth. Such conduits are ideal for the speedy delivery of misunderstandings, "fake news", and outright lies sent out as sound bites to test the worthiness, transmissibility, and impact factor of these packets of vaporware on the intended recipients. Periodic micro-insults, which only need sensitive recipient ears, will stymie the best-intentioned forward motion of a team. Once discovered, these subterranean tunnels must be plugged aggressively and declared unworthy of further human habitation, akin to clearing the wound of infection before healing may begin.

Number Three: Failure to Respect that Leadership Cycles Have a Natural Ebb and Flow

As Joseph Simone famously said "for academic leaders, the last ten percent of job accomplishment may take as much time as the first ninety percent, and may be not worth the effort." He then states that the average leadership duration should be 10 ± 3 years. Thomas Starzl reportedly said that surgical chair positions should have durations of 7 ± 2 years. We personally believe that the era of the chairmanship lasting until retirement is a dinosaur, like many of those who did such. New leadership at the Dean, Executive VP, or CEO levels are likely to bring in their own teams irrespective of the successes of the incumbents. Be prepared and try not to take it personally. In addition, it is important to have the insight that perhaps you no longer have the passion or institutional support to take your Division or Department to the next level. It is no service to anyone if you are just going through the motions, or as Rumsfeld says, "if you are coasting, you are going downhill."

In saying this, we comment that it is not a good thing to be constantly on the search for a better opportunity. There are no well-kept secrets in academic surgery and if a sitting chair is looking at another position, he or she must be willing to accept the brinksmanship that may result at home. Also, you probably will only receive one retention package. Your second trip to this particular well may result in a firm handshake and best wishes. Simone states that you should consider an academic move only if there is an improvement in anticipated environment and opportunity of 50% or more. The grass may look greener but when you get there the verdure most assuredly will not be luxuriant as once believed.

You will also be faced, as a leader, with faculty members who are constantly interviewing for another position. Often, they will tell you this during an early conversation after your arrival. Listen carefully, but make no promises or retention offers until you have done your due diligence as to the faculty member's value and track record of such claims. If the individual was an internal candidate for your position, listen even more carefully and gauge whether he or she will be an ally, or a passive or aggressive impediment to your vision (see Number Two, above). It may be best to cut the cord and allow them a graceful exit. Beware of faculty who announce that they have another offer, and a better one, as your first introduction to their job hunting. Michael Zinner wisely opined that anyone can have a first interview, or "first date", but once a second date is scheduled, it is appropriate and respectful to notify the chair.

Number Four: Failure to Remember that First Class People Recruit First-Class People; Second-Class People Recruit Third Class People, or as Rumsfeld Says A's Hire A's, B's Hire C's

The late William Longmire once commented that his secret to success as the first surgical chairman at UCLA was to hire great division chiefs and then get out of their way. Of course, he modestly simplified his success. We also later learned that this advice originally came from Theodore Roosevelt. Dr. Longmire provided his leaders with resources, support, and promoted them vigorously internally and nationally. He was neither afraid nor intimidated by their excellence. Michael Zinner, inarguably one of the greatest surgical leaders of our time, stated it this way, "learn to bask in the reflected glow." After all, it really does not matter who gets the credit as long as the job gets done well. Rikkers says it this way "leadership need not be lonely, wise chieftains grant authority and responsibility to those they had delegated assignments". Do not be afraid of hiring people who are smarter, more accomplished, or even better surgeons than you. Genghis Khan was an icon of political and military genius, but his greatest strength was in the ability to recognize and recruit excellent generals. Rikkers also state that the two most important roles of a leader are mentorship and recruitment. Mentorship leads to retention of those whom you have recruited. Rikkers also states truthfully that a lack of autonomy has been a driver for divisions of surgery to seek departmental status.

Saying this, you will make recruitment mistakes. We have made many of them and the senior author has often aggravated them by seemingly becoming an all you can eat buffet of second chances. After all, you put your pride and reputation on the line bringing in a physician or researcher who subsequently was found to be incompetent, dishonest, lazy, disruptive, or just a poor fit. Do your due diligence. The smallest red or yellow flag must be considered seriously, as should be its source. "Warm body" recruitments, especially in times of great clinical need, are to be avoided. Take your time, as removing someone from a faculty position can be extraordinarily time-consuming, litigious, and damaging. This is one of the reasons that we do not favor multiyear contracts to new recruits, despite their obligatory requests. We also believe that one should "excise the lesion" as soon as it becomes obvious that failure is present and a suitable attempt at rehabilitation is complete. Work with your human resources department and be prepared to keep meticulous records of interactions with the faculty member. Over the last two decades we do not believe that we have ever relieved a faculty member of his or her position without legal action being initiated.

Number Five: The Failure to Appreciate the Changing Priority of the Surgical Workforce

The failure to adhere to an occult progressive new paradigm of what's in it for me (WIIFM) will limit your impact unless you recognize that for some it is money, lifestyle and work/life balance that serves as the leading edge of the new practice model. We have had some practitioners look at us as though we had three heads when we wax prophetically about the pleasure and pain of caring for the sickest patient, the receipt of the hand-written note of thanks from a patient's relative, and the enduring pain that comes when surgical results are less than hoped and strived for- yet remain as indelible marks on your psyche. These are the best and the worst of experiences for a surgeon that defines us as human beings who are capable of a broad range of emotions. This is the life of service that prior generations thrived upon and that has created most medical advances. Although not the sole driver of some of those in medicine now, it remains as a powerful force that if unrecognized cannot be understood and utilized. If unacknowledged it will serve as a barrier as potent as the Berlin wall to any change. We implore you as the leader to take that difficult stand and face those pervasive issues in today's world with the ethical leadership that has defined medicine for the millennia. Remember to never forget that this is more than a job. Once it becomes a job then we are on a slippery slope for society and run the risk of merging with any of the multitude of occupations competing for the lead in the blind pursuit of financial bliss.

Number Six: Failure to Understand that the Leadership of Change Will Be Your Hardest Task

Machiavelli said that "there is nothing more difficult to take in hand, more perilous to conduct, or more uncertain in its success, and when you take the lead in the introduction of a new order of things." You were recruited to your new position because change was seen as necessary and you will be the driver and public face of that change. Hence prepare for criticism, inertia, and even insubordination from the few who are not willing to see the path ahead of them. The path is the key. Get your leadership team involved early, on the takeoff rather than the landing. Being crystal clear as you articulate your vision where your department, division, unit, or center should be is essential. Encourage feedback and be willing to amend, but never compromise on what is the right thing. Surgery is not a democracy.

If you do not have failures then you are not trying hard enough. If your shortcomings do not become visible then you are not out of your comfort zone and you are not growing yourself or your organization. If your true north tells you that something must change for the long-term goals of improved patient care and improved teamwork, then as Admiral David Farragut is oft quoted during the Civil War battle of Mobile Bay "damn the torpedoes, full steam ahead." Nothing should prevent your ethical leadership and moral compass from improving the lot of mankind, no matter how small an increment, as long as it is forward and with honorable intention. Should your effort appear to prove fruitless to those outside looking in, the reward is truly the learning experience from the failed process and further insight into oneself. That so-called "benefit" may initially be opaque and remain that way for the longest time; however, when it is least expected the learning might reappear as experience and guide in unexpected ways.

As Teddy Roosevelt so aptly stated "Far better is it to dare mighty things, to win glorious triumphs, even though checkered by failure … than to rank with those poor spirits who neither enjoy nor suffer much, because they live in a gray twilight that knows not victory nor defeat."

Be sure to join an organization that allows the new leader to create a new culture or pursue a worthwhile avenue, and in the process, understands that some changes take time and "mistakes", often made, must be recognized as part of the cost of doing business. You want to make sure that the organization is healthy enough that it does not adhere to the principle in which it is really easy to avoid all surgical complications by not operating at all!

A good salesman knows that the first thing to sell is yourself; the product (or vision or policies) are sold second. You must be clear, consistent, and above all honest first before expecting the right "others" to jump into the bus with you, or the wrongs to disembark.

A few quotes: General Eric Shenseki famously said "if you don't like change, you are going to like irrelevance even less." Rumsfeld says "dogs don't bark at parked cars" i.e. if you are not being criticized, you may not be doing much. Margaret Thatcher stated that "there is nothing more obstinate than a fashionable consensus. "Charles Darwin put this in evolutionary terms by saying that "It is not the strongest of the species that survives, nor the most intelligent, but the one most responsive to change."

Finally, remember that the place you landed was still standing when you arrived. They were doing some things right, including their decision to hire you. Do not throw the proverbial baby out with the bathwater. Build on the existing strengths and relationships even as you create your vision for new ones. Entire textbooks have been written about the leadership of change and change management. We have read quite a few and remember a little. Some of our favorites are placed in the reading list at the end of this chapter.

Number Seven: The Failure to Repeatedly Ask Yourself If What You Propose Is Fair, Is Clear for All to Understand, and Is What You Would Want for Yourself

This is the failure to ask yourself repeatedly if your message is appropriate for the task at hand or is simply the case of a square peg in a round hole. If so, it prevents the team from acceptance and rowing at the same cadence and in the same direction. The leader must be introspective at every step to understand who the team is, what it would like to become, and perhaps what it is capable of handling. As James Comey pointed out "doubt is wisdom." This should almost become a daily event and eventually will lead to a clearer understanding of the leaders' almost automatic response to a patient in distress, a family in need of consolation or any one of a number of crises and will ultimately reflect one's true north. Gates' rule number 32 is "never do anything to a patient you would not want done to yourself" also applies to the individual teammates. There will be many instances of external queries about the effects of change and your role within that organizational change. As long as one has been through the process of self-doubt, reflection and reassessment as to the true motivation beyond self, the leader will reconfirm the needed change and the wisdom to press on in the face of unstable times. The failure to anticipate those queries may derail your efforts but if the leader has done his/her internal measurement and homework ahead of time, then it will not be long before they are back on track.

Number Eight: Quitting Your Day Job

We can only hope that you did not enter medical school or complete a surgical residency with the ultimate aspiration of being a division chief or the chair of a department of surgery. (Even worse, if your primordial aspiration was to become a Dean!) Oh sure, you may have known that you were something special and a natural leader based on those glowing letters of recommendation received as an undergraduate and medical student. Nevertheless, your first and singular task was to learn how to be the best operating surgeon; one with expert technical skills, great patient empathy, and of course an intellectual curiosity. The days of the surgical chairman only occasionally operating with the help of a junior faculty or a fellow are now extinct, like their analogous dinosaurs. We have been visiting professors at a number of institutions where, when the Chair's surgical practice is mentioned, eyes roll and the conversation become funereal.

Even if you are one of those rare triple threat individuals with a funded laboratory and an international reputation, your junior faculty and residents need to see you in the Operating Room, blood and/or pus on your scrubs. This is especially true at night and weekends, as you must also take some call—and not the (once per month) "symbolic call" lorded over us by many senior egoist chairs at their multiple national meetings. Try to become an expert in one field and attain regional or national recognition in your ability to treat that disease surgically. It is difficult for a chair to have a busy tertiary practice with complex sick and often festering patients nowadays with all the administrative efforts and time sinks from the hospital and medical school. However, our 2 days a week in the operating room are usually our favorite and most rewarding days of the week. On the drive home, after a day in the operating room, one feels tired- an earned exhaustion. Compare that to the existential fatigue experienced after a day of meetings! Try to avoid having meetings scheduled late on your OR day or between cases so as to avoid any distractions. It is also important to scrub with junior residents, and be completely and utterly honest about your own complications at the surgical morbidity and mortality conference. In most cases you will be expected to be the grandmaster at this conference. Walk the walk.

A caveat: you will be watched, especially when new to the job. Other surgeons will wander through your operating room, seemingly to inquire how things are going or to wish you well, all in the subterfuge of really seeing how good you are as a technical surgeon. Like the cowboys of old, you must lead from the saddle. Be on time, get your own informed consents, and never malign the operating room publicly. If you are applying for a Chairmanship, insist on being Surgeon-in-Chief so as to be part of the solutions, not the problems, inherent in any academic operating suite.

Finally, do not appear aloof or unapproachable, even if you are busy and time conflicted. Make sure you sit in the OR lounge from time to time, telling a few bad jokes, but mostly listening on the fly to the concerns of all who work there. Host the departmental Holiday Party at your home and perhaps even a summer team-sporting event. When meeting with faculty, try to do so in their office. You can learn a lot by looking at the pictures and papers that adorn their walls. We have quarterly full Department meetings, and make sure a light supper is served.

This rule also applies because chairmanships may be ephemeral and you will need to rely on your hands and surgical skills if a change in leadership occurs. The ability to operate with skill and compassion will keep you employed, valued, and a candidate for other positions should this unlikely event occur.

Number Nine: Not Choosing Your Battles Wisely

You will be constantly faced with dealing with the urgent rather than the important. This is more than just time management; it is deciding where your scarcest resource, your time, is most effectively used. As a new chair your office will be flooded with faculty members with problems that have existed for years. You will be expected to solve these, in exchange for their undying trust and respect. (Don't believe it.) Listen carefully, but before you promise, do your homework. Be especially cautious if your predecessor is blamed for the problem's perpetuity. There is always more than one side to the story and usually a very good reason why this problem has been unsolvable for so long. Although getting a few quick wins under your belt is important, do not waste valuable energy or resources on the unwinnable or undoable. Sadly, these quick wins are often followed by a "what has he done for me lately?" Avoid the "tyranny of the urgent".

It is important to seek counsel of others. A "kitchen cabinet" or Division Chiefs meeting should be held regularly, at least monthly. Here, many of these skirmishes can be discussed with those who have longer institutional and departmental memories. Insist upon absolute confidentiality from these meetings, however, and be wary of, and confront early, any leaks. The Chair has a lonely job, so consider strongly hiring a deputy, or Vice-Chair, whom you can trust, and develop a succession plan for yourself and all of your leaders.

Perhaps a leaders' greatest strength should be "artful listening", as per Steven Sample. Your inner circle should be constructed on trust and understanding. You should assemble a team committed to what is best for the institution and the department, and be willing to exchange in free and often no-holds-barred conversation, in private. Disagreements should be encouraged, but a decision is made, all must support it as a team.

Early on, become colleagues and friends with your corresponding chairs of Medicine and Anesthesiology. You are joined with them at the hip clinically and academically. Larger battles, and those engaging your Dean or CEO, may result in a win, but also a loss of a precious ticket, as per Jerry Shuck. Choose these carefully and make sure they really benefit the greater good of your faculty or patients, as it may become a Pyrrhic victory.

Number Ten: Poor Management of Meetings and Committees

Someone once told us that a good week is when you have more cases than meetings. If that were true, we have very few good weeks. As a surgical leader you will have meetings and committees populating your calendar with evangelical abandon. Many of these you will need to attend, after all, you most likely will be the only one there representing the field of surgery, or having the voice of reason. Sometimes real money or resources are discussed; to be absent is to lose your turn at the till. You do not have to attend all of them, however. Be prepared, review the agenda, and if there is none, suggest that there be one at the next convening. Speak up and express your concerns, comments, or advice, but do not feel the need to interrupt every silence with your own words, unless they improve the silence. Occasionally take the opportunity to publicly complement another chair or department. (Not the dean, as to avoid appearing sycophantic). If in doubt as to the importance or necessity of the meeting, arrange for your Executive Assistant to page you 30 min into it, to allow for a graceful early exit, seemingly for an urgent clinical matter. For after hours' meetings, consider setting your smart phone to alarm 30–45 min into the meeting; you can always hit the snooze button if you want to stay.

The first consideration for your own meetings, according to Rumsfeld, is whether to call one at all. Can it be avoided with just a few phone calls or emails? Your direct reports are busy, as you want them to be, so be respectful of their time. Do not set a time or place that only works for your schedule. Send out an agenda, early, with time limits set for each item to keep all on track. If it is a regularly scheduled meeting, as with your Division Chiefs, invite agenda items, or at least have time allotted for open discussion. We strongly believe that no meeting should exceed an hour; 50 min is better. Do not let meetings be purely informational as that can be accomplished with just an email or document. Encourage discussion, even dissent, but keep things civil.

Start on time, and do not recapitulate for those who arrive late. It is disrespectful to the majority who were on time. Do not allow the use of smart phones by the attendees, unless it is to answer a call, and follow this rule yourself assiduously. Make sure everyone present is asked their opinion, and respect and explore differing views. Finally, the closing questions of any meeting should be: what was good or bad about this meeting, what have we missed, and what are the next steps? For the latter, assign responsibility. Avoid the formation of committees and subcommittees as a solution to a meeting's unsolved problems.

For individual meetings the two most common mistakes are surprise and location. If you ask to arrange a meeting with a faculty member, make sure they know roughly what it is about. No one likes surprises, and no one expects good surprises. If a formal meeting, such as one for evaluations, negotiation, or criticism, use your office. If informal, congratulatory, or just to check in, visit them on their home court.

Committee work is the bête noire of the academic surgeon. Remember that only about a third of committee members will actually work at it, whereas an equal proportion is "idiots and troublemakers" (Simone). The rest probably will not show up. If appointed or conscripted to a committee, try to be in that good 30%, despite the other claims on your time. When establishing committees, remember that less is more. In fact, like a cardiac arrest, their success is inversely proportional to the number of people in the room. Make them small, representing all stakeholders of the issue, and establish goals and a timeline.

Finally, it is all about time management. David Logan, of Tribal Leadership fame, says it succinctly: Don't let anyone commoditize your time. Here is a personal example: If paged, and I answer promptly, and I am then put on hold, I hang up (unless it is from a referring physician). Why? Well, when someone pages you they are essentially saying "stop what you are doing, and answer me now." If they cannot make themselves available for that return call, they are commoditizing your time. When you are re-paged, gently notify them of this simple rule of etiquette.

Number Eleven: Forgetting that You Need to Be More Catholic Than the Pope

The senior author's first academic leadership position was as Division Chief of General Surgery at UCLA. The laconic and underrated E. Carmack Holmes was my Chairman and mentor. Along with a lot of other good advice, he cautioned me to always be more Catholic than the Pope. In other words, you need to be above reproach in all matters clinical, ethical, and professional. The Department certainly had its share of outliers in those days, and he did not want his first leadership appointment to fall from Grace. Although I was initially affronted by this advice, I realized its importance early on, as I watched other surgical leaders, both at home and on the road, ignore it. Although some special dispensations or perquisites come with the leadership territory, they must be deployed with grace and humility, and as infrequently as possible.

This also means that you must expect this self-discipline from your direct reports and faculty members, without exception. Looking the other way for an individual, perhaps because of their busy clinical practice or grant funding, is an unforgiveable slippery slope. Needless to say, these conversations must be held in private, and documented. Chip Souba's classic, and factually based, article about Brock Star, a hugely profitable but disruptive cardiac surgeon, is an epitome of this caveat.

A corollary of this rule is the axiom: just stay put. John Cameron once stated that there were two kinds of Chairs, those who went to meetings, and those who took care of patients. It is important to go to regional and national meetings, and attain some leadership in them, but limit your time on the road as much as you can. Your faculty will most likely have limited travel time and money, and many silently (or not) resent your travels, especially if they are left covering your patients. Use national meetings to support your faculty and residents by nominating them to membership and committees. We personally do not attend meetings for over a two nights' stay, with rare exception. Chances are, if there is a black-tie event, we have already left the building.

Number Twelve: Poor Credit or Blame Assignment Mistakes

As mentioned earlier, learn to bask in the reflected glow of your faculty. The corollary of this was disclosed by Mike Zinner, when he said to not expect a lot of "thank you's" in return. It is difficult to sit at a meeting and watch someone take full credit for your work, or suggestion, or resources supplied, but it is best to stay silent. Forgive, but remember. Be generous with praise and credit, but beware those who begin to believe in their own press. To paraphrase Bear Bryant, if anything goes bad, you did it. If anything is semi-good, we did it. Finally, if anything goes really good, then they did it. Send emails out to the faculty publicly congratulating someone for a publication, or promotion, or acceptance into a surgical society. The obverse and deadly sin is taking the credit when it is not truly yours. A venal example of this is padding your CV with the work of your faculty.

For the most part, you should criticize in private and praise publicly, unless an act is so egregious that a rapid response is mandatory. Remember the words of Simone, "muck flows uphill … and fast" contrary to the laws of physics. In academics the leader must, at first whiff of a conflict, error, or other significant problem, avoid the response of burying one's head in the sand. Successful bullet dodging is rare. If you ignore it, it will not go away. Get the facts quickly for the rare horrendous surgical or research outcome, inform the Dean if necessary, and prepare a course of reparation. Consult your institution's legal team, and be wary of the press.

Number Thirteen: Failing to Keep Your Priorities

It is often said that the opportunity costs of leadership are precious, and usually include family and personal time. After all, these priorities often complain the latest, and the softest … until it is too late. This is the mistake we make the most frequently. The senior author has never left a position where he did not have a full bank of unused vacation days. His young children rarely saw him before noon on Saturdays, and unless they went to church, before noon on Sundays. These were his "catch up" days for writing and administrating. He was lucky to have a most understanding family, and still managed to attend almost all sporting events and dance recitals. Saturday night dinners out were a family tradition, although now we nearly empty nesters tend to have it delivered. But we know that we could have done a whole lot better except for ambition and ego, and it could have easily gone the other path of counseling, separation, and divorce. Make your family a top priority. Chip Souba wisely stated that "your family never reads your CV", and the old saw that no one ever lies on their deathbed wishing they spent more time at the office is a certainty. Try to go off the grid on vacations.

Do not fail to prepare for retirement, financially and personally. Maximize your pre-tax savings from day one. Have disability insurance. Counsel your junior faculty to do the same. Do not assume your health will be perfect forever, or that you can save for retirement after your kids finish college. Finally, do not ignore your own personal and spiritual health. Read, exercise regularly, and thank God every day that you have been blessed to be a surgeon.

Suggested Reading

Collins J. Good to great. New York: Harper Business Publishing; 2001.

Drucker PF. The effective executive. New York: Harper Collins Publishers; 2004.

Drucker PF. What executives should remember. Harv Bus Rev. 2006;84:145–52.

Goleman D, Boyatzis R, McKee A. Primal leadership. Boston: Harvard Business School Press; 2002.

Halverson AL, Walsh DS, Rikkers L. Leadership skills in the OR, Part I, communication helps surgeons avoid pitfalls. Bull Am Coll Surg. 2012a;97:8–14.

Halverson AL, Neumayer L, Dagi TFL. Leadership skills in the OR, Part II, recognizing disruptive behaviors. Bull Am Coll Surg. 2012b;97:17–23.

Kotter JP. What leaders really do. Harv Bus Rev. 2001;79:85–96.

Logan D, King J, Fischer-Wright H. Tribal leadership. New York: Collins Business Publishing; 2008.

Pearce LP, Maciariello JA, Yamawaki H. The Drucker difference. What the World's greatest management thinker means to today's business leaders. New York: McGraw–Hill; 2010.

Pearsall P. Toxic Success and the mind of a surgeon. Arch Surg. 2004;139:879–88.

Rikkers LF. Presidential address: surgical leadership-lessons learned. Surgery. 2004;136:717–24.

Rumsfeld D. Rumsfeld's rules: leadership lessons in business, politics, war, and life. New York: Harper Collins; 2013.

Sample SB. The Contrarian's guide to leadership. An Francisco: Jossey-Bass Publishing; 2002.

Simone JV. Understanding academic medical centers: Simone's maxims. Clin Cancer Res. 1999;5:2281–5.

Souba WW. Brock starr: a leadership fable. J Surg Res. 2009;155:1–6.

Managing Teams Effectively: Leading, Motivating, and Prioritizing Work

8

Justin B. Dimick

Introduction

The definition of what it means to be an effective surgical leader has changed. In the not-so-recent past, surgical leadership was synonymous with an autocratic, command and control style. This approach to leadership, which dominated for many years, often gave surgeons a bad reputation. Surgeons were often perceived as inflexible, tyrannical, and not "team players". There are clear advantages to the autocratic style (which are covered in other chapters in more detail), including getting things done quickly and strategically, which can be important when delivering surgical care.

However, the autocratic style of leadership is not the most effective way to lead a team [1]. The need to work in teams, and the collective intolerance of leaders who cannot work as part of a team, has banished most of those with the autocratic leadership style to the dark corners of most health systems. At best, the inability to work with a team severely limits one's leadership opportunities. At the worst, the inability to work with a team results in remediation, such as anger management, professional coaching, or even dismissal.

Teamwork has never been more important in the delivery of surgical care. Most clinical care is delivered by a multidisciplinary team of providers (e.g., breast cancer, bariatric surgery, transplant surgery). Quality improvement work can only be done by engaging all front-line staff (e.g., nurses, physicians, other providers) in a meaningful way. For surgeon-scientists, leading a team of researchers that bridges clinical and methodological disciplines is the only way to elevate your work to the level of sophistication that merits external funding in a very competitive environment.

J. B. Dimick (✉)
Division of Minimally Invasive Surgery, Department of Surgery, Center for Healthcare Outcomes & Policy, University of Michigan School of Medicine, Ann Arbor, MI, USA
e-mail: jdimick@med.umich.edu

© Springer Nature Switzerland AG 2019
M. R. Kibbe, H. Chen (eds.), *Leadership in Surgery*, Success in Academic Surgery, https://doi.org/10.1007/978-3-030-19854-1_8

Learning New Mental Models

Becoming a better leader often involves learning new mental models. Mental models are a useful way to make sense of complexity. In medical school, we spend many years learning mental models for various biological processes (e.g., trans-membrane receptors, T-cell receptors, etc…). These biological processes are no doubt much more complicated than the representations that appear in colored bubble diagrams in our textbooks. Nonetheless, it is widely accepted that this "working understanding" that comes from these mental models allows us to use this knowledge to benefit our patients, e.g., develop new medical treatments that can then be empirically tested.

In medical school and residency, we spend very little time developing mental models for understanding human behavior. A typical, but very simple, mental model that may be familiar to anyone who completed a surgical residency is "strong vs. weak". These simple mental models create a false dichotomy that can often be represented by proverbs, e.g., "actions speak louder than words". Leadership by proverbs is flawed, however, since every proverb has an opposite but equally correct proverb. For example, the opposite of "actions speak louder than words" is "the pen is mightier than the sword" (see http://www.rinkworks.com/words/proverbs.shtml) for a comprehensive list).

Leadership development is about learning more sophisticated mental models. Earlier in my career I served as the Associate Chair for Faculty Development in our Department and implemented an 8-month Leadership Development Program (LDP). Many cynics often ask, "What can you possibly learn from such a program that helps you become a better leader?". Although our data suggest there are many benefits, I believe the exposure to and learning new mental models was an essential component. In our program, we introduced mental models for leading change, working in teams, encouraging innovation, and many others. Combined with action-based learning projects, which provide an opportunity to try out and reflect on these new mental models, these programs can be powerful development experience.

Learning to effectively motivate and prioritize the work of a team are among the most important leadership mental models. In this chapter, we will discuss three models that each addresses an important aspect of managing teams. First, we will discuss the Fundamental State of Leadership and learn how to enter this mindset. Second, we will discuss how to effectively motivate and get the best from individuals on your team. Third, we will review a well-known framework for prioritizing work, but will reconsider it in the context of teamwork.

How to Lead Your Team

Many of the most common models of leadership focus on personality traits. Implicit in these models is the notion that by isolating and demonstrating the personal characteristics of a good leader we too can lead well. However, there is an alternative model promoted by Quinn and colleagues that stands in stark contrast to these trait-models of leadership. The Quinn model, which he calls the Fundamental State of Leadership, proposes that leadership is a state of being and not a set of traits— and each person leads best by bringing their unique self to a leadership role, rather than copying someone else's traits [2].

This model supposes that leadership is not a destination but rather a state that we enter and leave. This way of being is contrasted with our usual state in which we are comfort centered, externally directed, self-focused, and externally closed. Comfort centered means we adhere to our usual routine and shy away from activities that push us beyond what comes easily. Externally-directed means we are driven by what is expected from us and do not lead from our core values. Self-focused means we attend to our own needs without thinking about the larger goals of the organization, or those we serve. Externally closed means that we are not open to feedback and therefore do not see reality. Does this usual state sound familiar? Although it may be difficult to admit, it is where we spend most of our time. This state is normal and desirable for self-preservation.

However, when we transcend this usual way of being, we can enter the fundamental state of leadership. In the fundamental state of leadership, we are results centered, internally directed, other focused, and externally open. When we are results centered we can move out of our comfort zone and focus on ambitious goals that challenge us. When we are internally directed we are acting from our core values and not simply doing what others expect of us. When we are other focused we are sacrificing for the good of others and the organization—and we are putting their needs above our own. When we are externally open we are in a growth mindset in which we can accurately perceive reality and we are open to feedback.

Perhaps the best attribute of this particular mental model of leadership is that is not abstract philosophy—it is quite usable in every-day life. Quinn has proposed four simple questions to help you enter the fundamental state of leadership. When you are confronting a crisis, or a new opportunity, you can simply ask yourself these questions to help move towards this higher state of leadership (Table 8.1).

Table 8.1 Four questions to shift you into the fundamental state of leadership

By asking…	You shift from…	To…
Am I results centered?	Remaining in your comfort zone and following routine	Tackling ambitious goals and moving toward new possibilities
Am I internally directed?	Conforming to other's expectations and seeking external validation	Clarifying and living according to your core values with authenticity
Am I other focused?	Focusing on your own needs and success	Orienting activities based on what is good for the organization and the other individuals within it
Am I externally open?	Protecting yourself by ignoring feedback and not perceiving the environment accurately	Learning from feedback and perceiving environment accurately

How to Motivate Your Team

The science of motivating teams is fascinating because there is a huge gap between what the best scientific work shows and what we actually do in practice. In his book "Drive" Daniel Pink nicely reviews the scientific evidence behind motivating individuals at work [3]. The most common practice for motivating individuals is to pay for performance. If a leader wants more of a behavior, she will create financial incentives that reinforce that behavior. Unfortunately, the science tells us that this often does not work. Motivating with "carrots and sticks" does work but only for a narrow range of behaviors. The tasks for which incentives are appropriate are for simple, mechanical tasks where effort easily translates into productivity. However, in the current environment, where most tasks are cognitively complex and require innovative solutions, financial incentives do not work well, and can even compromise performance.

Numerous rigorous experiments on the psychology of motivation have found that monetary incentives do not work for cognitively complex tasks [3]. On reflection, these empirical findings are consistent with the challenges confronted by many surgical leaders, particularly in academic health centers. Motivating surgeons to be clinically productive is relatively straightforward. Offering large financial incentives—i.e., "eat what you kill" reimbursement models—predictably results in larger amounts of clinical revenue. However, other activities, such as academic output (e.g., grants and publications) are much harder to incentivize.

But there is good news: the science of motivation does provide a useful mental model for optimally motivating individuals on a team. There are three essential things that drive successful individuals: autonomy, mastery, and purpose [3].

- Autonomy: Our need to feel self-directed and choose our own work.
- Mastery: The opportunity to do something over and over again until we master it.
- Purpose: The sense that we are contributing to something greater than ourselves.

Providing team members with a sense of autonomy is essential. Human nature dictates that individuals are more effective when they chose their own direction. Practically speaking, this means making sure the team members want to be involved in a given activity or committee. When teams are made up of individuals who were assigned by someone else (i.e., did not choose to be there) they may have no sense of "buy in". As a result, they are much less likely to be effective on that team. Autonomy is not simply about control, however. Having a sense of control is important, but autonomy is more than simply choosing our own path. Matching individual team member's interests to their assigned tasks is critical. Of course, this means knowing what their interests are. A good leader will have a sense for what each team member's individual goals and interests are and can they match tasks accordingly. The best team leaders will have a running inventory of where each team member is hoping to grow, and therefore what they may want to get out of an experience.

Autonomy and mastery go hand in hand. As we discussed above, allowing team members to develop mastery over a skill set that matters to them is extremely important. The need to develop mastery—doing something over and over again until it comes easy—is one of the greatest drivers of human performance [3]. This is important in and of itself by giving us a sense of accomplishment. Mastery is the cornerstone of intrinsic motivation. This is apparent if you reflect on the zeal with which we all pursue our hobbies. But mastery of specific areas is also important for helping us achieve our professional goals. Once again, the team leader must appreciate the needs of the team members. A good leader has insight into which skills each individual is hoping to develop. A leader will also know what that individuals career goals are and will therefore know which growth opportunities will best help them achieve their individual goals. In a well-designed team, each member fulfills a role that will help them move toward mastery of something that is important to them.

The final key is to motivate your team to some higher purpose. Autonomy and mastery are important in and of themselves but work best when used to fulfill a purpose that moves us towards our vision. In surgery, and medicine, this is very easy. We all chose to become physicians because of this higher purpose—to help others. But sometimes we become distracted and take this mission for granted. Sometimes we just lose sight of the big picture. With expansion of new clinical service lines, we often talk about return on investment. When establishing new research centers, we talk about the papers and grants we will write. While this focus on the profit motive is prudent—"no margin, no mission"—it can be disheartening and lead to cynicism in the team. Framing these issues around serving some higher purpose—"no mission, no need for margin"—can connect these efforts to the true purpose, such as public benefits of new clinical programs, or the far-reaching impact of new research initiatives.

Communication is essential in establishing the higher purpose of an initiative. Practically speaking, this communication needs to be part of every meeting. Sharing the potential contribution that comes from achieving a shared vision needs to be communicated frequently. Often, teams and committees get caught up in the day-to-day work and forget the goals of their work. Starting each meeting by reviewing the long-term and short-term (e.g., of this meeting itself) is a way to ensure such ongoing communication.

Key Pitfall: Beware of Creating a Dumping Zone

This mental model stands in stark contrast to how we often think about assigning work as a leader: Delegation. Advice on leadership invariably includes the suggestion that leaders must effectively delegate in order to "leverage their talent" and become more efficient. Unfortunately, effective delegation is more complicated than this one-sided calculus suggest. The delegation must be a win/win scenario for the leaders and the individual or team being delegated to. The autonomy, mastery, and purpose mental model helps sort out whether a leader is delegating or simply dumping. The autonomy can be assessed by asking "Is this a task that the team members would choose for themselves?"; mastery can be assessed by asking "Will this project help the team members develop new skills that are in line with their goals?"; and purpose can be assessed by asking "Does this project clearly reflect the higher purpose of our organization in a way that is meaningful to the team members?"

How to Prioritize Your Team's Work

"What is important is seldom urgent and what is urgent is seldom important."
—Dwight D. Eisenhower

Appropriate motivation is important to get the most out of your team, but it is also important to make sure they are working on the most important tasks. Important tasks are those that best support the longer-term vision of the organization. Developing that vision and strategy are considered elsewhere in this book. Here we assume that these long-term goals are already known. Moreover, choosing the initiatives that are necessary to achieving this vision—i.e., tactical and strategic goals—are considered elsewhere in this book. This next mental model is about making sure these important goals get prioritized appropriately in the midst of the team's daily work.

Prioritizing work to achieve the long-term goals of an organization is an essential part of leading a team. A lot has been written about prioritizing work, but the most widely cited mental model is Steven Covey's classic two-by-two table, which is sometimes referred to the Eisenhower Matrix (see the quote above) or the Urgent/ Importance Matrix [4, 5]. This mental model considers two essential attributes of a team's work, whether it is important (vs. unimportant) or urgent (vs. non-urgent) (Fig. 8.1).

Fig. 8.1 The Urgent/ Importance Matrix

	Urgent	Non-urgent
Important	I Critical activities	II Important goals
Not important	III Interruptions	IV Distractions

One of the keys for using this matrix effectively is to understand what is truly important and what is really urgent:

- Important: These are activities that are essential for achieving the future goals (i.e., vision) of your organization.
- Urgent: These are activities that demand immediate attention.

These two attributes placed in a two-by-two table create four quadrants (I–IV). To prioritize a team's work, the leader needs to be constantly evaluating which quadrant the team is working in at all times. Quadrant IV represents those tasks that are non-urgent and not important (i.e., distractions). Examples of distractions are the lengthy discussions about last weekend's football game, many of the phone calls and emails that we receive, or "checking" Facebook. Clearly team member's time should not be spent in this quadrant. Similarly, quadrant III represents issues that are not-important but are perceived as urgent (i.e., interruptions). Many teams may spend a good deal of time on both distractions and interruptions. A good team leader will recognize when this is occurring and reprioritize and reorient the team's work.

While the distinction between what is urgent and what is not urgent may be straightforward, it is more difficult to identify what is truly important for the team. As discussed elsewhere in this book, the ability to understand which tasks are most important relies on knowledge of the desired future state the team is working towards—i.e., the vision for the organization. Quadrant I tasks include the important, urgent work and represents where most of us spend our time, i.e. "putting out fires". These tasks are by definition important to the team and aligned with the vision of the larger organization. For a surgeon, quadrant I tasks obviously include unplanned clinical care, such as reoperations for complications. These are clearly important and immediately shift all other priorities—no matter what they are—to the back burner. Dealing with complications falls under our very important long-term goal of being a good doctor. But it should be recognized that if most of the time is spent in this quadrant, less attention is spent on the tasks that support our most important longer-term goals (quadrant II).

Good strategies for limiting quadrant I activities are essential. Of course, any practicing surgeon cannot completely eliminate unplanned clinical care. But it can be limited with a more controlled clinical practice, either by having scheduled shifts of clinical activity (e.g., trauma or acute care surgery) or by having a lower morbidity elective practice (e.g., minimally invasive surgery). Perhaps this is why many surgeons slow down their clinical practice, either the volume or the complexity, when they take on administrative roles where they bear more responsibility for long-term goals (e.g., chief medical officer, department chair, etc…). A leader would not be very effective if they were missing all of their important meetings or did not have the necessary cognitive energy to address the complex problems that come with such roles. Recognition and explicit consideration of this trade-off is important for every leader.

It is also important to recognize that not all quadrant I activity is not unplanned clinical care. There are numerous administrative "fires" that need putting out. These require time and attention but may not be explicitly tied to achieving our vision. The key strategy for addressing these is prevention. Chances are that many of the quadrant I activities could be eliminated by carefully focusing on quadrant II activities. We can likely prevent many of these crises by developing our productive capacity and paying daily attention to our long-term goals. Personality conflicts among team members are a frequently occurring example. Identifying and addressing these potential conflicts early, through team building and relationship building, can keep the team focused on quadrant II tasks.

Most of our teams need to spend more time in quadrant II, completing the non-urgent but important tasks. Stephen Covey calls this "*putting first things first*" [3]. These tasks usually represent two key domains. First, they represent tactical and strategic goals of the organizations. These tasks answer this important question: "What things if done differently would allow us to achieve our vision?" Second, these tasks represent ways to build our production capacity. They answer this important question: "What things if done differently would allow our team members to grow in a way that improves their productivity?". While the former group of activities may be obvious, the second are often not. A classic example of overlooking the investment in production capacity that is highly relevant to this book is leadership development. This short sightedness is captured in the following exchange:

CFO asks CEO: "What happens if we invest in developing our people and then they leave us?"
CEO: "What happens if we don't and they stay?"

If we honestly reflect on how we lead teams, we probably spend more time than we should addressing emergencies and don't spend enough time working towards our most important organizational goals. Dealing with emergencies has a gravitational pull, especially for surgeons. We chose our specialty because we all crave immediate gratification. We live for small, bite size, fixable problems. Achieving long-term goals requires us to break the pull of these activities. Determining the future direction of an organization—setting the vision—is a key skill in leadership, but prioritizing your team's work to achieve these goals is just as important.

Key Pitfall: Try Not to View All Non-urgent Communication as Waste

It is important to recognize that as humans we do enjoy interacting with each other in social ways. And this is not a bad thing. Indeed, many of these Quadrant III and IV distractions could actually be filed under "building relationships" among co-workers. These social ties create empathy among team members and enhance our sense of fun at work. This justifies many of the game rooms and fun spaces that characterize many modern offices. Only the completely rational and super-efficient *homo economicus* would edit out all of these interactions. If we reflect for a minute, I am sure someone comes to mind for all of us. Is that person a good leader?

Probably not as good as they think they are. But this is clearly a fuzzy line and a zone of high rationalization, where we can justify excessive chattiness and Facebook indulgence. A good team leader can help bring this line into better focus. This line is clearly crossed when distractions and interruptions get in the way of the organizations goals.

Summary

Leading teams effectively has never been more important for surgeons. Providing multidisciplinary clinical care, building collaborative research efforts, and engaging front-line personnel to address quality problems all rely on top-notch team leadership. Learning to effectively lead, motivate, and prioritize the work of a team are among the most important mental models for optimizing team performance. The fundamental state of leadership provides a practical set of questions for stretching beyond our usual state of being and improve our team leadership. The science of motivation provides a useful mental model for optimally motivating individuals on a team, ensuring each team member has a sense of autonomy, mastery, and purpose. The Urgent/Importance Matrix provides a useful framework for prioritizing teamwork, reminding us to eliminate distractions and interruptions and spend enough time on non-urgent important tasks that help us achieve our long-term goals.

References

1. Tannenbaum R, Schmidt W. How to choose a leadership pattern. Harvard Business Review, May–June 1973, No. 73311.
2. Quinn RE. Moments of greatness: entering the fundamental state of leadership. Harvard Bus Rev. 2005;83:74–83.
3. Pink DH. Drive: the surprising truth about what motivates us. New York: Riverhead Books; 2009.
4. Covey SR. The 7 habits of highly effective people. New York: Free Press; 2004.
5. The Urgent/Important Matrix: Using Time Effectively, Not Just Efficiently. http://www.mindtools.com/pages/article/newHTE_91.htm.

How to Manage Difficult Team Members

9

Nathaniel J. Soper

Introduction

The punch line for a much-repeated joke about surgeons is, "Oh that's God; he's just pretending to be a surgeon". The unique demands on surgeons—the ability to act decisively even when data are limited, the necessity to improvise when unexpected situations occur, and excellent eye-hand coordination—created somewhat of a mythical aura about surgeons. Surgery as a profession has also long been closely linked to the battlefield and the armed forces. Up until the late twentieth century, these historical influences reinforced the so-called 'surgical personality', one which is overbearing, hierarchical, and frequently treats subordinates in an abusive manner. Given the dictate for 'managing the ship' of the operating room, the need for quick compliance with orders and intolerance of delay reinforced these attributes, and the behavior was tolerated. Increasingly, surgical leaders are called upon to manage teams in meeting rooms and the C-suite. It has become clear that the best surgical decisions and outcomes are associated with good teamwork and a flattening of the hierarchy within a surgical team, both inside and out of the operating room. This concept has been reinforced with introduction of crew resource management techniques into the operating theater, 'sign-ins' which introduce all participants to one another, 'time-outs' to identify potential errors in the making, and an acknowledgement that all members of the team should have the ability to 'stop the line' should problems occur. Self-defining characteristics of surgeons—to do what is necessary within time constraints, to project a calming confidence under stressful conditions and the ability to rise to the occasion are still necessary and reinforce good leadership principles, but the brash and arrogant caricature is no longer necessary nor desired.

N. J. Soper (✉)
Northwestern University Feinberg School of Medicine, Chicago, IL, USA
e-mail: nsoper@nm.org

Nevertheless, and as in all areas of human interaction, multiple personality types exist in the surgical environment. Within a group—team, section, division, department or task force—many different personalities exist and need to be managed effectively by leadership to accomplish tasks. These personality types, when carried to the extreme, may result in 'difficult' or 'disruptive' members of the team.

Numerous different classification systems attempt to categorize personality types. One such system is the Meyers-Briggs Type Indicator®, which identifies 16 specific types of personalities. Each of these types has a different outlook on life and way of dealing with issues. From the leader's standpoint, when hiring decisions are being made, the underlying personality of the individual must be taken into consideration. An incredible curriculum vitae and stellar list of accomplishments are enticing in a potential recruit, but a personality that doesn't mix well with the culture of the existing team is a recipe for disaster. Background and reference checks specifically asking about interpersonal interactions are important when considering a new hire, as one of the most time-consuming, and least productive, aspects of a leader's job is moderating disputes among team members who 'can't play together in the sandbox'. A bad hire costs an incredible amount of time, energy and money to undo.

For those in leadership positions, it is important to understand the local institution's by-laws on rules governing behavior—most state words to the effect that practitioners must "adhere strictly to the ethics of their ... profession, to work cooperatively with others ..." and that the member may be considered for removal were he or she to act in ways that ... "are believed to be detrimental to patient safety or inconsistent with the efficient delivery of patient care" (Northwestern Memorial Hospital Bylaws). Finally, leaders should understand that if team members cross the line into the category of 'disruptive' that all subsequent dealings with the individual should be documented and records be maintained for future considerations.

'Difficult' Team Members and a Leader's Response

Multiple different personality types will undoubtedly populate any team or group of which one is a member. Leaders must learn how to best manage these personalities within such groups. The appropriate management style is necessarily dependent on the situation, the number of people in the group, and the group's purpose. A leader must rely on his or her emotional intelligence and experience to navigate these sometimes tricky personality waters. In Chap. 6 the concept of emotional intelligence was explored. The leader may need to call upon self-awareness, social awareness, self-regulation and, certainly, social skill in dealing with the difficult team member. Furthermore, as discussed in Chap. 4, there are at least six leadership styles that can be invoked in any given situation. It has been said that a successful leader will use the different leadership styles as a professional golfer uses the clubs in the golf bag, choosing a club based on the demands of a particular shot, i.e. situation [1].

There are several specific personality types that may negatively impact a team. Those with difficult personalities have developed their personal traits over years and generally learn that they can wear down others to ultimately get what they want. The leader must identify the individuals' personality characteristics, realize the ways in which these attributes may complicate the functioning of a team, and learn techniques that may temper the expression of these traits. Some of these specific personality types include the following: The passive-aggressive personality type may undercut the leader's authority by sniping, using sarcasm, and engaging in non-playful teasing. These individuals generally don't like being the center of attention, however, and don't like open confrontation. A strategy that may work with them is to redirect their attention to the issues rather than to other team members, and ask them to come up with specific action items to contribute to the team's activities. A second, easily recognizable personality type is the chronic whiner ('Eeyore'), who sees the glass as always half empty, points out the difficulty in every opportunity and blames others for every problem that arises—"I told you so" is their common refrain. The leader must stay positive, but realistic, with these individuals and be quick to point out positive outcomes from decisions made by the team. Diametrically opposed to the negative personality types are those who always try to please others, over- committing themselves and unable to give an honest opinion when the observation is not positive or popular. The leader must only very carefully delegate tasks to these individuals, help them learn how to say 'no', and specifically call them out to give candid opinions when the facts are unfavorable. There are also those who are unresponsive and disengaged and who refuse to reveal their true motives. They often will not participate voluntarily in a formal meeting and reveal little about themselves. These people must be drawn out to participate in group meetings, asking them open-ended questions and listening closely to their responses. Finally there is the traditional 'surgical personality' who is hostile, abusive, domineering and arrogant. These individuals can engage in bullying activities and must be treated differently than the remainder of those mentioned above. If disruptive behavior is manifested in a group meeting the individual should be excused from the meeting with a subsequent private and transparent discussion of the inappropriateness of the interactions.

As a leader, it is important to understand that each of us has the capacity to demonstrate some of the above behaviors on any given day. The expression of our personalities may be impacted by events taking place in our personal lives or in other arenas—leaders must work diligently to not allow these extrinsic factors to negatively impact their dynamics with members of their team. This requires emotional intelligence and the targeted ability to blunt one's own emotional responses.

The basic reaction of a leader to the aforementioned difficult individuals is not to take the interactions personally and to realize that you really cannot change the underlying personality type. What you can change is your response to the individual, your attitude toward them, and your behavior. Remember that for others, too, an untoward personal situation may underlie the personality type being expressed and empathy can sometimes be used to de-escalate an explosive situation. Make it clear that you respect the individual, but you also expect to be treated with respect in return. One highly charged word that should probably be avoided during a difficult interaction is 'attitude'—this is a subjective term and the leader should instead focus on the behavior of the individual. Ultimately, the leader must try to understand the different personalities existing in one's team and learn to manage to their strengths.

Disruptive Team Members

The difficult personality types referred to above can slow down progress within an organization and give the leader headaches. However, a different class of difficult team members is that of the disruptive member who must be specifically identified and managed separately. The term *disruptive physician* is defined as those who exhibit abusive behavior that "interferes with patient care or could reasonably be expected to interfere with the process of delivering quality care" [2]. Lucian Leape has described many different examples of disruptive behavior [3]. When reading through the specific behaviors characteristic of disruptive physicians, many match the definition of the 'surgical personality' of old. These behaviors include outbursts of anger, throwing instruments, demeaning behavior, sexual comments or innuendo, negative comments about other physicians' care, but may also include unethical or dishonest behavior. These disruptive behaviors are associated with an increased likelihood of errors by the healthcare team [4]. Behaviors of this nature make those around them try to avoid the disruptive physician, hesitate to make suggestions about patient care or deflect their attention away from the patient. This disruptive behavior also has a potent negative effect on morale within the healthcare team, making life for others around them, particularly those lower in the pecking order, miserable and more likely to disengage. Disruptive behavior has been shown to be associated with higher turnover among nursing and technical support staff in the medical setting [5]. Disruptive behavior by surgeons is thus associated both with worse patient care and higher healthcare costs.

Surgical leaders must strive to identify disruptive team members and deal with them firmly but appropriately. The identification of these individuals can be complicated by those around them being intimidated and not wishing to draw attention to themselves by such reporting. Disruptive behavior may be identified in online event tracking systems, by unusual events described in the Morbidity and Mortality system or during a sentinel event disclosure. Gerald Hickson and his group from Vanderbilt have written extensively about the identification of problematic disruptive physicians by their association with increased numbers of unsolicited patient complaints [6].

Whereas the interpersonal behavior of all people may lapse from time to time, it is estimated that approximately 3–5% of physicians demonstrate persistent patterns of disruptive performance [6]. These disruptive outbursts occur most frequently in high stress areas of the medical care environment, such as emergency departments, intensive care units and operating rooms. Not infrequently, these behaviors may be tolerated because the individual is a clinical rainmaker. Once a disruptive physician is identified, however, there must be a clearly defined response. Leaders must promote excellent care in an environment that fosters quality. They need to understand, develop, and implement fair, reliable processes for addressing questions about behavior, performance and outcomes [7].

The first goal in addressing disruptive behavior is to truly understand the situation by obtaining enough event-related data to ascertain reliability. Certain behaviors cannot be tolerated whatsoever—these include sexual harassment/misconduct or discrimination based on gender, race, religion, sexual preference or gender identification. However, there are always two (or more) sides to any story. If there has been a single unprofessional incident, an informal 'cup of coffee' conversation is the most reasonable reaction by leadership or by someone designated by the leader [8]. This conversation informs the individual that the behavior was both noticed and was unprofessional and does not adhere to the team's standards. The individual should be asked about events or situation in his or her life that may be impactful and can be addressed. Recurring patterns of disruptive behavior must be handled with more formal interventions. The short term goal is to help the disruptive team member achieve insight into the negative aspects of his/her behavior. The long term goal is to restore professional conduct and eliminate the disruptive behavior.

Recurring negative events require a more formal response. Hickson's group has developed a pyramidal, tiered, system of intervention that starts with a level 1 "awareness" intervention when recurring unprofessional events are identified [7]. I believe it is the leader's role to be directly involved, usually solo, at this stage. At this meeting the data suggesting the pattern of disruptive behavior are discussed in order for the individual to gain insight into his/her actions, and a clear expectation of altered behavior is expressed. After the meeting, a letter is written to the disruptive surgeon outlining the purpose and outcome of the meeting, and a copy is placed in the employment file.

If the awareness intervention does not have the desired results and a pattern of disruptive behavior persists, the situation is elevated to a level 2 "guided" intervention by authority [7]. I have found it helpful to involve the hospital's Chief Medical Officer in a formal discussion with the offender at this stage of intervention. This meeting must be carefully planned out in advance, keeping in mind your desired outcomes/objectives and the talking points that will be addressed by each person. Usually, the disruptive individual is referred for evaluation in our physician wellness program to assess for underlying causative factors (such as marital issues, substance abuse, burnout, etc.) and/or for psychological assessment and counseling (e.g. anger management interventions).

Finally, should the individual show no change in his/her behavior, level 3 intervention is required, which is a disciplinary action that follows organizational policies and procedures [7]. The resources of the institution are brought to bear at this point, and may ultimately lead to restriction of duties or dismissal, with reporting to the appropriate governmental agencies.

It is mandatory that throughout this process adequate records are maintained that document the progressive steps. Remember that there are at least six potential audiences for any such written records: the physician under review, the physician's attorney, future leaders of the healthcare system, the defense counsel, the judge, and the local newspaper. Disciplinary action with formal investigations and a reporting to the National Database is the least favorable outcome and all attempts should be made to restore the disruptive team member to a good professional standing.

The Impaired Team Member

The term 'impaired' has been defined by the American Medical Association as a disability resulting from psychiatric illness, alcoholism, or drug dependence. The prevalence of these impairments in physicians is likely equal to or greater than that of the general population given they are often associated with fatigue, stress, and/or easy access to drugs. Impaired fitness for duty may also accompany the burnout syndrome. Burnout can lead to depression, substance abuse and even suicide [9]. There are no good studies assessing the incidence of physical illness among practicing surgeons, and surgeons are not immune to cognitive and/or technical decline with aging [10]. When all of the above conditions are considered, it is estimated that one quarter to one third of all physicians will experience, at some time in their career, a period of time during which they have a condition that impairs their ability to practice medicine safely [3].

Physician leaders must bear in mind that unusual or disruptive behavior may be the outward manifestation of impairment in a surgeon, be willing to confront the issues rationally, and be aware of the local resources for investigation and management. Impaired physicians usually are identified by those around them noticing unusual or atypical behavior. Per hospital by-laws, a urine or blood test for alcohol and/or drugs may be ordered immediately. Most physician health programs mandate the impaired physician to undergo a treatment program with subsequent routine monitoring as a condition of reinstating hospital privileges and medical licensure. When returning to active practice after a period away, the surgeon should be entered into a focused professional practice evaluation system with close monitoring during the first few months.

Identifying the team member, particularly a surgeon, whose physical or mental capabilities have declined due to aging, may be difficult. Many surgeons are passionate about their profession and have not developed interests outside of the hospital and so resist the concept of retirement. The majority of health systems do not have mandatory retirement ages nor do they routinely assess competence as physicians age. Part of this laissez-faire attitude may be due to concerns about age discrimination-related legal actions. Should concerns be raised about a surgeon's competence due to aging (or any other cause of physical or mental decline) the individual should undergo testing to assess both cognitive and manual skills functions.

Conclusions

Academic leaders must work with multiple personality types. These include team members whose personalities have the potential to interfere with team dynamics. The leader must learn how to deal with difficult team members, utilizing emotional intelligence and various leadership styles. The traditional 'surgical personality' can no longer be tolerated in today's team-based health care. The leader will occasionally be called upon to deal with truly disruptive, or impaired, surgeons and must be familiar with the various options open to them for effective management of these difficult situations.

References

1. Goleman D. Leadership that gets results. Harvard Bus Rev. March–April 2000.
2. Federation of State Medical Boards of the United States, Inc. Report of the special committee on professional conduct and ethics. Dallas, TX: Federation of State Medical Boards; 2000.
3. Leape LL, Fromson JA. Problem doctors: is there a system level solution? Ann Intern Med. 2006;144:107–15.
4. Benzer DG, Miller MM. The disruptive-abusive physician: a new look at an old problem. Wisc Med J. 1995;94:455–60.
5. Rosenstein A. Original research: nurse-physician relationships: impact on nurse satisfaction and retention. Am J Nurs. 2002;102:26–34.
6. Hickson GB, Federspiel CF, Pichert JW, et al. Patient complaints and mal-practice risk. JAMA. 2002;287:2951–7.
7. Reiter CE III, Pichert JW, Hickson GB. Addressing behavior and performance issues that threaten quality and patient safety: what your attorneys want you to know. Prog Ped Card. 2012;33:37–45.
8. Rosenstein A, O'Daniel M. Impact and implications of disruptive behavior in the perioperative arena. J Am Coll Surg. 2006;203:96–105.
9. Patti MG, Schlottman F, Sarr MG. The problem of burnout within surgeons. JAMA Surg. 2018;153:403–4.
10. Trunkey DD, Botney R. Assessing competency: a tale of two professions. J Am Coll Surg. 2001;192:385–95.

How to Effectively Manage Up

10

Gerard M. Doherty

Introduction

Managing Up is often misunderstood. This concept for those in management positions can be confused with "sucking up"—insincerely positive behavior intended to be observed by the manager's superiors in order to curry favor—also known as being an apple-polisher, teacher's pet, brownnoser, sycophant or toady. The point of Managing Up is not to impress one's superiors, but rather to recognize and perform well in those parts of your role as a manager that support the superior.

Leadership positions in academic surgery are complex, and even successful leaders are not uniformly effective across the spectrum of their challenges. However, one of the ways to fall far short of expectations, and to fail to realize one's potential in areas of strength, is to ignore the importance of Managing Up. Leaders must recognize that they are a part of someone else's team, in addition to building their own. They need to recognize what is expected of them, and how to perform in ways that support the goals of their superiors. This includes the goals that the superior has formally set, as well as the ones that they have not recognized.

Succeeding in Managing Up can include many types of behavior, and may require specific actions for specific manager/superior relationships. However, a few principles are important. All successful strategies in this arena include most or all of these (Table 10.1). Your goal in this arena is to become the indispensable partner that your boss cannot imagine doing without.

G. M. Doherty (✉)
Brigham and Women's Hospital, Dana-Farber Cancer Institute, Harvard Medical School, Boston, MA, USA
e-mail: gmdoherty@bwh.harvard.edu

© Springer Nature Switzerland AG 2019
M. R. Kibbe, H. Chen (eds.), *Leadership in Surgery*, Success in Academic Surgery, https://doi.org/10.1007/978-3-030-19854-1_10

Table 10.1 Principles of
Managing Up

Make time to meet
Trustworthy and loyal/private sounding board— public support
No surprises
Offer solutions/provide options
Do boss's homework first and best
Never bypass the boss
Know the boss's perspective for key goals
Know boss's strengths/Compensate boss's weaknesses
Float the boss's trial balloon

Principles of Managing Up (See Table 10.1)

Make Time to Meet

As a leader in a department of Surgery, it is easy for you to become completely booked with meetings and focused on the important projects for the department. It is surprising how suddenly long stretches of the year can slide by. It is absolutely critical that you as a department leader make, and insist upon, time to meet with your superiors.

During the meetings, it is critical to provide updates on important projects, and to inquire about institutional initiative and plans. However, it is also important to leave some time unstructured to explore areas that are not sufficiently mature to have made it onto a "to-do" list. It is essential to have an institutional perspective to guide the department in ways that best contribute to the whole. You cannot get that perspective without one-on-one conversations.

In any meeting, pay attention to the last 5 min. Whether the meeting lasts 20 min or 2 h, it is common that an issue introduced right at the end is the most important information. This is when one of the parties may finally bring up the topic that they promised themselves to mention.

Trustworthy Private Sounding Board and Public Support

Trust is critical to a strong working relationship at any level, but especially in leadership. As an important part of the institutional team, you should be both constructive and supportive. The institutional leaders should be assured that they can count on you to maintain confidentiality and to understand the importance of "the cone of silence" for discussing ideas that may ultimately not be implemented [see: https://en.wikipedia.org/wiki/Cone_of_Silence_(Get_Smart)]. In those discussions, you should be willing to be critical, or to play devil's advocate, for the proposal. Sometimes these discussions can be animated, though criticisms should never be personal. The discussion must then remain within the leadership group; a lack of discretion will be followed directly by being left out of the next conversation.

Once a decision is made, however, you must publicly support the plans; the alternative pathway of active opposition to a major issue is often resignation. Dissent outside of the decision process can undermine the implementation process for a plan that the institution has adopted. You take the path of dissention at the peril of the institution, the department and your role. It is disruptive for other members of the department to observe this, and may undermine their commitment that is fundamental to department success.

Your commitment to behave in this way can be difficult in some circumstances. However, to remain central to the decision-process of the institution and to avoid undermining department goals, you must be viewed as a trustworthy colleague who will provide well-considered criticism in private, and strong support in public.

No Surprises

Surprises are great for birthdays, but constructive institutional reactions are built around anticipation. Particularly if there is the potential for bad news, then you should alert the institutional leadership at the earliest possible moment. It is not necessary for all details to be confirmed in this situation. A "heads-up" call followed by a subsequent reassurance is far preferable to a surprise disaster.

Offer Solutions/Provide Options

Leaders are in place in part to anticipate and recognize problems. It is frequent that leadership meetings are centered on addressing some problem or challenge.

When you bring a problem to institutional leadership, it is always necessary to bring at least one recommended course of action. It is preferable to bring a variety of 2–3 options with strengths and weaknesses, including costs, attached. It is never sufficient to bring only the problem, and to anticipate that the solutions will come from the institutional leadership. Even if the resources for the proposed solutions must come from the institutional level, rather than the department, the proposal should come from you as the person who presents the challenge.

Do Boss's Homework First and Best

Special projects delegated from one's boss are usually an imposition. Being asked to run a search committee, lead a curriculum review, or chaperone a strategic planning process is rarely an opportunity that is on your wish list. The project may not contribute to the department goals for the year. The time to meet these new targets has not been anticipated in your plans. However, there is very little option to refuse a project assignment, and no real option for putting it off or doing it poorly.

It is perfectly reasonable to accept a project and to note that you will come back with some ideas on the necessary timeline and resources. However, once the project has been offered, then it must be completed, and it must be done well. This is not just because it is the boss's project. Presumably, the project has important institutional implications, if the institutional leadership has decided to commit some of your time to it. Taking the project on and then doing it poorly, or late (which often go together) does a disservice to the institution and indirectly to your department members.

You should make this project a priority for your own team. Assign some of your best assets to supporting the work. Set an aggressive timeline internally, and get started right away. The opportunity to support the institutional agenda outside of your direct workflow is an important one for both you and the institution.

Never Bypass the Boss

Your boss has a boss. That may be the hospital board, the university president, or some other hierarchy, but everyone reports to someone. It may be tempting at times to go around your immediate institutional leadership to achieve some goal that has been stymied through your usual channels. However, bypassing the boss in this way will likely undermine the remainder of your relationship.

It can be hard to take no for an answer if that stops your progress in an area important to you. Going around your boss to try to get another answer will poison your relationship. In order for them to do their job well, they need to know that you will respect their position. If you are asked to go around the hierarchy by your boss's supervisor, you should first let your boss know of the approach and the goals. They may wish to be involved, or may choose not to do so, but your openness will be positive for your relationship. If your boss's supervisor asks you not to involve your boss, then you are on very fluid ground (quicksand) and should do your best to save yourself.

Know the Boss's Perspective for Key Goals

You have annual, shorter term and longer term goals. It is critical that you understand the priorities of your supervisor with respect to these. Which goal is the most important to them? Which goal is nice but optional? Which annual goal is a critical opportunity this year, and which one could be deferred to next year without penalty?

Goals are important as they guide our actions through the year. Many goals are only partially achieved, or not approached at all due to other circumstances. As the year progresses, you are faced with decisions about which goals to prioritize and which to postpone. If you do not have a clear sense of which goals are important to your institutional leadership, then you may learn at the end of the year that you have chosen to work on the goal that does not best contribute to the institutional progress. Sometimes this is straightforward, but often it is not. Working through the decisions as the year goes along, in regularly scheduled meetings, will avoid surprises on both ends.

Know Boss's Strengths/Compensate Boss's Weaknesses

A part of your role as an "indispensable" partner is to complement the weaknesses and strengths of your colleagues. Everyone has areas of performance in which they excel. Your supervisor may be an expert at building clinical programs and affiliating with outside institutions, but may be bored and ineffective at human resources and compensation plans. You need to recognize that and take advantage of the strengths, while helping them to avoid working in the areas of weakness.

This is not as difficult or deceitful as it sounds. Within a short period, you will understand both the strengths and weaknesses—your boss may even tell you what they are. Then you can look for areas of their strength where you need help, and use their expertise. The weaknesses may be no less obvious, but can be trickier to support. The option of avoidance is fine—do not ask for help with HR issues from your finance expert boss—but you still must avoid surprises and keep them informed. More likely, they will avoid the areas where they are not as skilled. If they are particularly insightful, they may take your advice directly when you offer to help with one of these areas.

Float the Boss's Trial Balloon

Your boss has goals, and they are not always straightforward or easy. Likely, they are more elaborate and dependent upon the actions of others than yours are. In the pursuit of those goals, your boss may have some things that they need to try out—either on a smaller scale in your area, or to be developed by a group within the institution. Your boss needs someone responsible to work through these issues with them in ways that will not necessarily appear to be their failure if the project does not work.

You can be a very useful surrogate by serving as the project leader or trial site for these ideas. If the project is a success, expect the boss to take credit, but know that you have made yourself an indispensable part of the team. If the project fails, then you will not be penalized within your direct group since this can be positioned as an institutional imperative. By performing in this role, you help your supervisor to explore ways to address their goals without taking all of the risk directly.

Conclusion

Managing Up comes naturally to those leaders who recognize that every boss has a boss, and that we are all a part of someone else's team even as we build our own. Empathy for your supervisor—recognizing the world as she or he sees it—will help you to employ the principles delineated here, and to become the indispensable team member that we all aspire to be. Below are case studies that provide examples of common scenarios that involve successful and unsuccessful Managing Up strategies.

Case Studies

Case Study #1: Do Boss's Homework First and Best

A Department of Surgery chair was in the third year of his tenure when asked by the medical school dean to lead the search committee for the next chair of Obstetrics and Gynecology. He quickly assented, and drew on his prior experience as a member of two search committees to determine how to proceed. However, it was September, and he had a full schedule of work for the Fall. He was recruiting faculty members for his own department, preparing for committee meetings at the ACS Clinical Congress, completing an editorial project, and continuing to try to build his practice. At his monthly meeting with the dean in mid-October, he had a suggested slate of committee members to invite, which they revised together, and he invited them. The committee first met in the second week of November to determine an advertising, communication and recruitment plan.

By the time the first candidate files were submitted, the holidays became an obstacle for campus visits. The committee had had four meetings, with little to discuss at each, and one of the leading candidates ultimately withdrew after not visiting the campus because the recruitment process at a rival institution was moving more quickly. The search committee chair was surprised to find that by mid-January, the only viable candidate that they had was the internal division chief from the obstetrics service.

In their January meeting, he expressed his concern to the dean, who responded, "I know—it's a hard job. Don't worry, I won't ask you to do it again."

From a Dean's perspective, one of the most important pieces of work in any year is filling gaps in campus leadership. The delegation of such an important component as leading a search committee is a dangerous opportunity for the committee chair. The Surgery chair in this case failed to recognize that this position had to either be a high priority and done expediently and well, or the request should be denied (also at the chair's peril). In reality—the only option is to accept the request, and then make it a high priority for the Surgery department staff.

Case Study #2: Know the Boss's Priorities for Key Goals

A division chief had been promoted to the role from within the department. She had made her reputation on her research successes and funding for a SPORE program in her field. She had her initial goal-setting meeting with the Department of Surgery chair soon after her promotion, and received guidance on the chair expectations of RVU targets, research productivity and teaching responsibilities.

At the 6 month mark, they met again to review the interval performance. The division chief was very proud of her achievements: the members of the division had submitted three IRB applications, two R21 and two R01 applications. They had publications in press, and abstracts to be presented at upcoming national meetings. To achieve this, she had instituted an internal "mini-sabbatical" system that provided 4 weeks free of clinical work for faculty members preparing an R-level grant. However, they were 20% below their projected clinical productivity.

To her surprise, the department chair was livid. Though the research productivity was excellent, the clinical productivity would not generate sufficient funds to pay the division expenses including faculty salaries. He was concerned that she had created an expectation among her group that the highest priority was research work, and that there was no responsibility to meet their revenue-generating targets.

In this case, the division chief has failed to understand the department chair's priorities in their mutual goals. She was supposed to increase the research output of her division, but she could not do that at the expense of clinical revenue generation. If her plan was to lose money for some period of time as an investment in expanding the research program, then that should have been explicit from the beginning with both the department chair and her faculty members.

Case Study #3: Compensate for the Boss's Weaknesses

A department chair known for his decisiveness and willingness to make hard decisions had a problem. He had two valuable senior faculty members who were competitive with one another, one of whom had been recruited to his department along with her clinical group, which included her husband. The rivalry between the two senior faculty members had become personal, and had led to accusations of research duplicity against her. An investigation showed that the allegations were not supportable, but the process left her disgruntled with her department and chair, and in search of a new position.

The chair's general approach to problems was head-on. He scheduled meetings with the two senior faculty members to try to resolve the animosity. He offered additional resources to support the work of the offended person, to keep her from leaving. He met with her repeatedly to ask what resources she needed.

However, his department administrator recognized that this effective chair's strength was directness, which would not work in this case. He had little patience for the "softer side" of management. The problem in this case was not resources, and the two senior faculty members were never going to back down from their mutual dislike. She recognized that her boss would not understand the emotional issues in this case, nor the importance of the family dynamic of moving to take this job, and potentially moving again. She suggested that he meet with the offended faculty member's husband to discuss the effects of another potential move on the family and their joint careers. By changing the conversation from one of purely professional circumstance to a broader outlook of the effect on the family, and the career of the "trailing spouse," the chair was able to retain the program.

In this case, the administrator was able to help her boss accomplish something outside of his natural skill set (Compensate for the Boss's Weakness), by recommending a course of action that she knew he would not recognize on his own.

Case Study #4: Floating the Boss's Trial Balloon

Academic departments have complex missions; of the three major ones (clinical, research and teaching), only the clinical work is easily and regularly measured. One department chair wished to have quantification as clear for research and teaching as she had with RVUs (relative value units) for the clinical work. She charged two division chiefs with developing a system to count the time and effort put into research work (funded and unfunded), teaching and administrative effort. She specifically wanted a measurement system that could quantify these efforts.

The two chiefs spent 3 months of careful work reviewing systems used in other departments, interviewing faculty members and making smaller presentations of portions of the plan. When the full plan was presented to the faculty, there were substantial objections to it based upon the amount of effort that would be necessary to keep track of all of the activities. With the opportunity to gauge the full faculty reaction to the plan, she was in position to back away from it, rejecting the idea that the faculty would spend all of their time making journal entries. The plan was never implemented, though the chair was careful to thank her two division chiefs publicly for exploring this on behalf of the department.

In this case, both the chair and the division chiefs did their jobs well. The division chiefs were willing to be the point people on the chair's project, and to bear the criticism of the proposal (Float the Boss's Trial Balloon). They enabled the chair to explore and ultimately reject the plan without having it be her direct setback. She used the division chiefs to evaluate this approach, and expended a lot of their effort on it, but in the end rejected the work-product rather than the people.

Suggested Reading

Abbajay M. Managing up: how to move up, win at work, and succeed with any type of boss. Hoboken, NJ: Wiley; 2018.
https://hbr.org/2015/01/what-everyone-should-know-about-managing-up. Accessed 19 Sept 2018.
https://www.tinypulse.com/blog/what-does-it-mean-to-manage-up4. Accessed 19 Sept 2018.
Managing Up. Harvard business review 20 minute manager series. Boston, MA: Harvard Business Review Press; 2014.

Conflict Resolution: How to Successfully Manage Conflict

Sandra L. Wong

Introduction

Management of workplace conflict is critical if teams and organizations are to continue to grow and accomplish their core missions. The nature of healthcare systems is increasingly complex and everyday work done around patient care, personnel management, and payment reform creates tension across all the key stakeholders. Conflict in this environment is inevitable and leadership in academic surgery demands the ability to feel comfortable with conflict and the ability to come to successful resolution. By nature of the skills needed to manage conflict, elements of management principles, tenets of communication and difficult conversations, and negotiation are woven into this review and discussion.

There are four major types of conflict: relationship, task, process, and status [1]. Conflicts can have elements of more than one type and rarely do major conflicts fit squarely into a single category. Identifying a root cause may help with conflict management and resolution. *Relationship* conflicts are simply defined as "a clash of personalities," or a personal disagreement. This type of conflict can be hard to manage when egos and a desire for control lead to parties feeling disrespected and hurt. More subtle causes include personal insecurity which can have an extreme manifestation as habitual victimization. Relationship clashes at work [2] range from denial ("I don't see any issue here") to aggression (bullying behavior) and can also encompass many variations of passive-aggressive behaviors.

Efforts to increase self-awareness, coupled with empathy and compassion in the workplace are examples of effective tools for dealing with relationship conflicts. When members of the same team have a long history of disagreement or dislike, that dysfunctional relationship needs to be addressed in order for the team to

S. L. Wong (✉)
Geisel School of Medicine at Dartmouth, Hanover, NH, USA
e-mail: Sandra.L.Wong@dartmouth.edu

© Springer Nature Switzerland AG 2019
M. R. Kibbe, H. Chen (eds.), *Leadership in Surgery*, Success in Academic Surgery, https://doi.org/10.1007/978-3-030-19854-1_11

succeed. Strategies for resolution include giving the parties an opportunity to hear each other's point of view. Possible pitfalls include ensuring that such actions to unite do not have unintended consequences of worsening the situation by either worsening the divide or by worsening how the conflict is perceived or managed by leadership.

Beyond personal disagreements, there are three other types of well-defined workplace conflict. *Task* conflict is a common source of disagreement at work and typically results from a dispute over a task or project. Different agendas and different goals (or even the perception of different goals) exacerbate these types of task conflict. *Process* conflicts are disagreements about how things are getting done, rather than what the work is. There can be overlap with task conflict, but one distinguishing characteristic is whether the conflict is over the outcome (task conflict) or how the decisions are made (process conflict). *Status* conflicts commonly manifest over who is "in charge" or who deserves credit for work being done.

Causes of Conflict

Causes of conflict can be attributed to opposing positions, competitive tensions, or emotion (e.g., egos, power struggles). There may be a tendency to think of conflict in very stark terms: enemies and allies. This mental mindset, in and of itself, speaks to emotion as one of the major underlying causes of conflict. In many so-called rivalries, emotion can trump data and reason, making even small gaps seem like large chasms. Further, gaps in communication can cause and/or exacerbate conflict.

Why It Is Important to Manage Conflict

In practical terms, non-relationship conflicts arise with power struggles (titles, money, resources) as well as status (influence, credit or attention) despite the relatively hierarchical structure of surgery departments and health systems. The disruption that accompanies such conflict may have implications for access and productivity, quality of patient care, revenue, workplace dynamics, and the ability to perform cutting-edge research at academic medical centers.

Conflict Management Styles

Conflict Avoidance

Lack of conflict management is tantamount to doing nothing [1]. Avoiding conflict, especially over a long period of time, leads to conflicts that fester, eventually growing to resentment. Employees often withdraw and confidence in leadership erodes. Unfortunately, this outcome is not only avoidable, but also potentially very difficult to detect because these employees or groups are not usually in crisis. A common scenario is one in which the team or teams underperform. Conflicts appear to be resolved but they are merely dealt with on a very superficial level, with a shiny veneer masking real issues. Occasional attempts at resolution, ironically, can be met with unease because of disruption of a stably unstable environment.

Not managing conflicts may not be disruptive in the short term, and in fact, many leaders who tend to avoid conflict may be competent, well-liked and highly collaborative. However, managers who "do not manage" eventually have to deal with problems of accountability and underperformance [3]. Ultimately, the desire to be well-liked and a so-called team player can lead to ineffectiveness and possibly heighten team tensions because trying to make everyone happy often backfires. Learning to be comfortable with conflict is often coupled with understanding that few people actually like conflict, but leaders must be willing to deal with conflict and have difficult conversations rather than skirting major issues.

The bystander effect has been described as a contributing factor to why some longstanding conflicts remain "open secrets." Employees who observe problems were far less likely (and possibly less willing) to speak up if they thought their peers observed the same issues. A set of studies [4] on the impact of the psychological phenomena of the bystander effect were conducted. When employees believed they were the only ones privy to an issue, they were 2.5 times more likely to raise the issue. The "diffusion of responsibility" among a group appears to morph into individual responsibility, and importantly, these findings were robust even when controlling for factors such as psychological safety (safety to speak up) and perception of whether speaking up would have an impact. These results have several implications for leaders. They emphasize the need to encourage open communication since leaders may, by nature of the position, be somewhat removed from the everyday discussions and be "in the dark" about issues unless they are specifically brought forward. Assumptions may be made that "everyone knows," when that is in fact not the case. Specific to leadership in clinical departments and hospitals (especially with leaders in new roles) are important issues around clinical competency, substance abuse or other health problems, and harassment.

Escalation of Conflict

Elements of self-management are necessary when taking on leadership roles. Employees expect leaders to lead and model courageous behavior, especially in times of conflict. There are times when "picking your battles" may be appropriate and a decision to avoid a minor issue is made. To be sure, harmony in the workplace should be valued, but there are times when conflicts surface and must be addressed. To that end, disagreement and debate may be favorable, though clearly, fighting is not.

While fighting certainly increases tension in the workplace, harboring tensions, emotions and misunderstandings also create tension, and ultimately leads to isolation, hopelessness, and burnout at the individual level. The balance between conflict avoidance and conflict seeking [1] must be calibrated. Escalation of conflict is the end result if conflict is not managed/resolved. Unwillingness to address conflict, or conflict avoidance, creates a true negative energy expenditure which is associated with a less productive, less effective workforce.

Elements of Healthy Conflict

On the other end of the spectrum, it is important to note that conflict can be a favorable characteristic of high performing organizations, and managing conflict in this context can actually strengthen collaboration and increase creativity and innovation. In fact, strong leaders do not fear conflict and see the positive side of conflict. Many understand the inevitability of conflict and seek it out, possibly to recognize and better understand the various stakeholder perspectives of a complex organization.

Healthy conflict must be rooted in a healthy environment, one in which parties do not have fear of criticism or penalty when engaging in honest conversation. Lack of trust in a work environment creates a lack of psychological safety and potentially controversial ideas are never surfaced. This is a missed opportunity for learning, discussion and constructive feedback.

In the current healthcare environment, teams are increasingly deployed to address complex problems, whether it be interprofessional teams around patient care (e.g., disease site management teams in a cancer center) or physician-administrator dyads or workgroups for the daily management of clinical operations. A misdiagnosis of why teams underperform often leads to efforts that are actually workarounds to managing the root cause of why collaborative efforts fail—unresolved conflict. Such workarounds, or even deliberate actions to improve collaborations such as team restructuring efforts, can actually increase points of conflict.

Further, recent efforts to improve employee engagement in organizations may have the unintended consequence of exacerbating conflict avoidant behavior with downstream consequences of decreased productivity and, ironically, increased employee burnout. Davey [5] posits that conflict becomes "a dirty word" in the modern workplace and is viewed as antithetical to teamwork, engagement and a positive culture at work. As a result, so-called "conflict debt" builds up because difficult decisions are deferred.

Principles of Conflict Management

Tools that allow for the effective management of conflict can be transformative not only for morale but for productivity, moving conflict from the liability column to the asset column. It bears stating that urgent situations call for an entirely different approach and there may be times when negotiation principles are not appropriate when conflict arises. Leaders need to be prepared to make quick decisions (e.g., crisis management) when there are life-threatening, legal, or other critical moral/ethical imperatives.

Assessing the Situation

There a several key steps to take when analyzing conflict, ideally prior to taking any action [1]. First, *seek to understand the involved parties* (including yourself), including management styles and how styles may or may not match. This may be a particularly relevant step if the conflict is outside the department or with unfamiliar parties. Then, *identify the type of conflict* to help understand the underlying cause of the conflict. *Determining your goal* or what you hope to accomplish helps to determine the final step, which is to *decide how to act*.

Major options for action range from doing nothing (or walking away) to taking action (including indirect or direct action). Assessing the situation allows time for preparation and preparation often includes consideration of multiple strategies which may be important if the situation is very fluid or potentially highly emotionally charged.

Preparing for Conversations

Some conflicts need to be resolved expeditiously. If a situation is likely to fester, then more immediate resolution allows for a more proactive and less reactive approach. Some particularly egregious situations demand attention and even a notice of intent to have a conversation will set expectations and prevent rapid de-escalation while allowing all parties to "take a (much needed) breath."

When time allows, preparation for potentially difficult conversations can lead to better management of emotions and set expectations for conflict resolution. In fact, having upfront discussions about communications styles can be helpful even in advance of have a more conscious approach to conversations. For example, leaders with a very direct communication style may want to convey that early on in work relationships in order to avoid unintentional miscommunication.

Preparation for any potentially difficult conversation takes stakeholder perspective and organizational context into account. Anticipating different scenarios may be particularly helpful in managing one's emotional response to conflict and ensuring that the conversation does not get derailed because of emotions or because a relationship conflict is allowed to compete with or take precedent over a critical issue. Additionally, taking communication tips into account can help maintain a fluid conversation.

Approaches to Conflict

When conflicts arise, it is easy to fall back on personal managerial styles, which may either be linked to a fierce desire to win ("hard positional bargaining") or a desire to maintain the relationship at any cost ("soft positional bargaining") [6]. When those taking the hard line are in negotiation with those pursuing a soft bargaining position, an agreement is often reached, but the result is often not the most optimal outcome, though likely most favorable for the hard positional bargainer who has dominated the conversation with threats and demands for concessions. The scenario with two soft negotiators is likely to result in resolution since a premium is placed on building and maintaining relationships, offering concessions and avoiding confrontation. However, the outcome may also not be the most optimal, as illustrated by the O. Henry allegory "The Gift of the Magi" in which the characters Jim and Della each sell their most treasured asset in order to buy a gift for the other, with Della selling her hair to purchase a chain for her husband's gold watch while Jim sells his watch in order to buy beautiful combs for his wife's hair.

One can imagine the scenario with two "hard liners" as the most difficult to manage and as the one in which resolution may not come to be. A better route to conflict resolution is needed. Decades of work from the Harvard Negotiation Project and the classic "Getting to Yes" book [6], which focuses on principled negotiation methods. The underlying basis of this approach can be summarized in four basic points: *(1) separate the people from the problem; (2) focus on interests, not positions; (3) invent multiple options looking or mutual gains before deciding what to do; and (4) insist that the result be based on some objective standard.* Mutual respect and understanding become the focus and this may be particularly applicable when there is time for a cooperative approach. This approach leverages overarching principles such as valuing relationships, managing emotions, active and emphatic listening to identify interests and options. These tactics can inform approaches to conflict resolution (Table 11.1).

Indeed, emotions do drive decisions and often result in getting entrenched in positions. This is why positional negotiation so often leads to unresolved conflict. Managing the emotional aspects of conflict is critical, especially in forming a needed basis of trust. Just as redirecting from personal tensions to the conflict at hand (separating people from the problem) serves as an effective strategy, turning

Table 11.1 Negotiation skills can translate to conflict resolution

Principled negotiation element	Tactics	Strategy for conflict resolution
Separate people from the problem	Understanding all stakeholders' perspectives can decrease misunderstanding (conflict is rarely one-sided)	Often, the problem is not created by people, but people need to work together to resolve the problem
Focus on interests, not positions	Engage in active listening; Strive to understand motivations and goals	Asking "why" can help get focus on interests and not positions; Decreases reliance on emotion (which can contribute to blame and criticism)
Invent multiple options looking for mutual gains before making a decision	Understand facts in the context of needs, interests, and goals	Express and discuss strong emotions to increase understanding of all stakeholders' perspectives
Insist the result be based on an objective standard	Yield to principle, not pressure	Acknowledge and be acknowledged; reason and be open to reason

Adapted from Fisher et al. [6] and Mind Tools Content Team (www.mindtools.com) [7]

the focus away from positions to interests can move key stakeholders beyond an impasse. Understanding the root cause of a conflict may require precisely defining the issues around which there are conflict. Once the issues are clear, it is important to separate the positions from interests.

Positions are "stands" that are taken on issues while interests are those underlying concerns which can be affected by how the conflict gets resolved. Many unresolved conflicts end at an impasse because positions are viewed as irreconcilable differences. However, positions ("this is what we stand for") do not always mirror a party's interests. Conversations that seek to understand and reconcile underlying interests create value and opportunities for successful resolution of the conflict. Key components include (1) taking time to ask "why" in order to help get focus on interests and not positions and (2) expressing and discussing strong emotions in order to increase understanding of all stakeholders' perspectives.

Communication Tips to Encourage Resolution

Two aphorisms come to mind when the topic of effective communication is raised. Commonly, it is not what you say, it is how you say it. And, secondly, it is often not what's said, but what's heard.

While it may be too simplistic to simply say that a change in tone would solve all communication problems, it is important to remember that perceptions of tone are exceedingly difficult to discern with nonverbal communication. Email correspondence, so common in the current work environment, is a good reminder that words do not always translate to the same message when written vs. when spoken. Indeed, being heard is not the same as writing a long email and expecting that the entire message, while memorialized, is read and properly interpreted. Further, those who have difficulty with phone conversations (again due to the paucity of nonverbal communication (specifically body language and eye contact) that is lost even though elements of a party's tone is retained) are advised to meet in person if possible.

Having a productive conversation is hard when it starts with language that can be perceived as an attack [7]. Conversations that begin with a perceived accusation often never really become a true conversation because the response starts in a defensive mode, essentially preventing either party from focusing on the issue at hand and possibly creating escalation. Effective "nonviolent communication" skills emphasize "honestly *expressing*" and "empathetically *listening*" as the two major components of the model. Nonviolent communication places a focus on better communication [8].

There are four steps of the model: observations, feelings, needs and requests (Table 11.2). Articulating *observations* of the conflict should be done without judgment or evaluation. Stating how the observation makes one *feel* leads to *needs* that are connected to the identified feelings. Feelings should include very specific behaviors can be acted upon whereas statements about hard personality traits tend to be less actionable, especially in the workplace. The last component is a very specific *request* related to the observation.

Table 11.2 Communication strategies for conflict resolution

Four steps for "nonviolent communication"	Conversation examples	
	Rather than…	Try this
Observations	"You did X, Y and Z…" or "You are (insert personality assessment)"	"When I see you do X, Y, and Z…" (use specific observations of behaviors)
Feelings	"and that behavior is not acceptable…"	"it makes me feel (insert emotion)…"
Needs	"and it needs to stop happening at any meeting"	"and I need…"
Requests		"Would you (insert action item)?"

Adapted from The Center for Nonviolent Communication. https://www.cnvc.org/learn-nvc/the-nvc-model [8]

The model is a two-way conversation, with the other party poised to *consciously* receive the information in the same four pieces. In this manner, elements of the conversation are more likely to foster compassion rather than conflict. Intentional listening skills help to mitigate feelings of under-appreciation that can trigger strong emotions as well as lead all parties to be acknowledged during the conversation.

Many other conflict resolution models or tips can be applied. While out of scope, there are specific strategies for dealing with frequently seen scenarios involving passive-aggressive behavior, deep-seated anger, and bullies. It may be helpful to discuss several pitfalls in conflict management and review possibly helpful solutions [1].

As a leader dealing with a conflict, your team may become upset and disengage (or in a worst case scenario, they mutiny). Understanding the underlying cause, and acknowledging it, is the first step in resolving and repairing the relationship. Ultimately, the group's confidence will need to be earned back. Conversely, there may be a situation in which a conflict arises with one's boss. Because of the reporting relationship, the resultant emotions of anger and fear are at odds. Consider the following steps: cool down, show respect, focus on business, and clearly explain intent (or the issue at hand) when discussing the conflict.

Understanding the Impact of Management and Conflict Resolution Styles

Rather than strictly dealing with or managing emotions, which tend to fluctuate with environment/context, understanding how managerial styles impact conflict resolution styles may provide a more effective framework for improving communication and engaging in more effective conflict resolution. What individuals' managerial styles help codify are strengths and weaknesses, as well as a better understanding of what motivators and stressors are. A very effective use of this is a better understanding of how your style tends to interact, either synergistically or at odds, with others' styles.

Table 11.3 How conflict approach styles interact

	Avoider	Seeker
Counterpart is an avoider	• Lean toward inaction/Doing nothing • Feelings and emotions are hidden	• The conflict seeker is aggressive in demanding concessions (possible solution: manage the degree of bullying) • The conflict seeker may behave passive-aggressively (possible solution: use active inquisition to encourage active participation in the conversation)
Counterpart is an Seeker	• The avoider worries about preserving the relationship (possible solution: be direct about feelings and needs) • The avoider may get bulldozed (possible solution: identify common goals)	• It may be a contentious discussion (possible solution: be alert to the pitfall and manage emotions) • Neither party is afraid to speak up, risking saying things that neither party truly believes or intends

Adapted from Gallo, A. HBR Guide to dealing with conflict. Boston: Harvard Business Review Press, 2017 [1]

Recall the stark contrast between conflict seekers and conflict avoiders (Table 11.3). In this example [1], anticipation of conflict styles and directed consideration of stakeholder perspective can help the parties prepare for the conversation and work toward resolution. One can imagine that the tactics around a conversation between two conflict seekers would be quite different than if it were two conflict avoiders. Further, a greater appreciation of one's own management and communication style leads to greater self-awareness and improved self-management. Those who value relationships and collaboration will need to be better about infusing objectivity and confronting conflict when working with those who are motivated by action and results. The latter can seek to be more patient and empathetic in order to improve discussions with the former. Team engagement exercises that include style inventories can create a better work environment and, ultimately, set the stage for better identification and management of conflicts.

Conflict Resolution

As stated, results or decisions must be based on objective criteria. Successful resolution of a conflict results in (1) satisfying as many interests as possible, (2) a result that feels fair and reasonable to stakeholders, and (3) ends with intact relationships among the parties.

Once a resolution is in place and executed, it may be sensible to "make rounds" or do regular check-ins to ensure sustainability. Borrowing the Plan-Do-Study-Act (PDSA) cycle from healthcare improvement scientists [9], the "study" phase of the PDSA cycle includes close observation and learning from the consequences of the "plan" itself. Notably, further modifications ("act") to the plan itself may be necessary to document and maintain change.

For teams, the ability to learn from conflict resolution itself should be considered. Proverbially, "don't waste a good crisis") and reap the benefits of the process of conflict resolution (including increased understanding; self-awareness/insight; team dynamics and cohesiveness). Having a retrospective look at the points of tension can lead to more efficient and proactive behaviors going forward.

Non-resolution of the Conflict

What if there is a failure to resolve the conflict? There may be severe consequences when conflicts are not resolved. From a business perspective, there may be a loss of productivity and downstream impact on access to care and net revenues. More broadly, organizations may experience increased barriers to collaboration as trust issues go unresolved. There may be a stifling of creativity and innovation, with impact on the effectiveness of the team and possibly of the composition of the team itself if employee retention becomes an issue as a result of a changing or unsupportive work environment.

Re-exploring options is critical at this juncture. Consideration of asking for a "third" position or mediator may lead to success if there is agreement to ask for and use help and if there is an agreement to consciously work together toward resolution. Forcing the use of a third party, especially if it invokes the reporting structure (organizational chart), may only serve to exacerbate a conflict and may create downstream consequences in an academic setting. If there is a deliberate determination to "walk away," that intent needs to be clearly stated. If there is a need to "cool down," making this a temporary hold, all parties need to recognize the potentially volatile issues leading to such an exit. If there is truly an impasse, take the time to commit to exploring other possible solutions (e.g., going from a win-win scenario to the so-called BATNA, or best alternative to a negotiated agreement) [6]. If the conflict continues to escalate, avoid cycles of action and reaction. In other words, remain calm and avoid escalation by refusing to react.

Can Conflict Be Prevented?

Some tenets for preventing or decreasing conflict include strategies such as setting expectations (communication) for acceptable behavior. Leaders may seek to recognize and understand various stakeholders' perspective. Unearthing productive conflict can reap big rewards. In healthcare, many missions of a medical center appear to be at odds with each other: Value vs. volume. Standardization vs. innovation. Actually working through these tensions is not only necessary, but can result in improved productivity for the department and health system.

Looking for conflict is not the same a picking a fight. Preemptively "looking for" conflict can often serve as a litmus of the workplace environment and can help decrease gossip and resentment. A buildup of resentment has heavily detrimental effects in the long term so earlier detection and proactive resolution can pre-empt bigger problems downstream. Being on the lookout for conflict can actually help with early recognition of issues before they bubble up to the surface. This may be particularly true if there is concern that the work environment has not engendered enough of a "safe community" to allow for such conversations.

Preserving and encouraging productive conflict allows people to speak honestly, express disagreements, negotiate different viewpoints, and work under a certain amount of pressure. Conflict in this light is positive, fostering innovation and creativity, disrupting complacency, and actually instilling a sense of accomplishment [10].

Generational Conflicts

"Generational issues" in the workplace are often discussed in the context of cross-generational differences and conflicts [11]. While differences across generations are a known entity, Millennials (born between 1981 and 1996) are most frequently discussed because this group comprises the vast majority of medical students, trainees, and (now increasingly) junior faculty in academic Departments of Surgery. Interestingly, what examinations of the workplace have demonstrated is that Millennials on a team are different from one another. Avoiding the pitfall of pigeon-holing or stereotyping Millennials on the basis of age is the first step to decreasing generational conflict. In fact, that same pitfall holds true for aging surgeons as well, remembering that there is no rationale for misunderstanding an entire generation. Principles for addressing conflict apply across generations, recognizing that age and rank in an organization does not necessarily inform a single approach to conflict management. The commonality across generations is a true need to feel valued on the job and a desire to contribute to the organization and its mission despite less flattering characterizations that Millennials switch jobs frequently, desire a flat work environment, and a better work-life balance than their older colleagues.

Conclusion

Conflict in the workplace is inevitable and are categorized into four main types: relationship, task, process, and status. Some degree of conflict can actually be beneficial to organizations by disrupting complacency and by fostering innovation and creativity. Conflict management is a key leadership skill and demands the ability to feel comfortable with conflict. Specific skills are helpful when managing conflict, and include elements of management principles, tenets of communication and difficult conversations, and negotiation.

References

1. Gallo A. HRB Guide to dealing with conflict. Boston: Harvard Business Review Press; 2017.
2. McKee A. "Why we fight at work," HBR.org, June 13, 2014. https://hbr.org/2014/06/why-we-fight-at-work.
3. Hussain I, Tangirala S. "Why open secrets exist in organizations" HBR.org, March 18, 2019. https://hbr.org/2019/01/why-open-secrets-exist-in-organizations.

4. Hussain I, Shu R, Tangirala S, Ekkirala S. The voice bystander effect: how information redundancy inhibits employee voice. Acad Manag J. 2018; (epub ahead of print).
5. Davey L. The good fight: use productive conflict to get your team and organization back on track. Vancouver, BC: Page Two; 2019.
6. Fisher R, Ury W, Patton B. Getting to yes: negotiating agreement without giving in. 3rd ed. New York: Penguin Books; 2011.
7. MindTools. Essential skills for an excellent career. https://www.mindtools.com/pages/article/newLDR_81.htm.
8. The Center for Nonviolent Communication. https://www.cnvc.org/learn-nvc/the-nvc-model.
9. Institute for Healthcare Improvement. Tools: Plan-Do-Study-Act (PDSA) Worksheet. http://www.ihi.org/resources/Pages/Tools/PlanDoStudyActWorksheet.aspx.
10. Lovric D, Chamorro-Premuzic T. Too much team harmony can kill creativity. HBR org. June 28, 2018. https://hbr.org/2018/06/too-much-team-harmony-can-kill-creativity.
11. Davey L. The key to preventing generational tension is remembering that everyone wants to feel valued. HBR.org, July 16, 2018. https://hbr.org/2018/07/the-key-to-preventing-generational-tension-is-remembering-that-everyone-wants-to-feel-valued.

Change Management: How to Effectively Lead a Cultural or Organizational Change

12

K. Craig Kent

Introduction

One of the most daunting but ever present challenges for any leader is change management. Why are humans so fixated on remaining the same? The responsibilities of a complex job are many and can be overwhelming; this is particularly true for physicians. These responsibilities can be initially daunting but we eventually grow accustomed to the challenges of our environment. We devise effective ways to succeed in stressful environments and eventually develop routines. Moreover, we are provided resources to facilitate our success and become accustomed to these resources whether they be salary, support staff or space. Then a leader comes along, perhaps you are that leader, and a decision is made to diminish resources or increase expectations or productivity or for that matter just change the status quo. The routine is disrupted and there is the need to adapt. Sometimes change means working harder or differently, or there are fewer resources, or a new direction that does not align with original vision. Change can also result in a more positive environment, increased alignment, or even enhanced resources. In many cases it is a mixture of both. Surprisingly, even positive change for some can be disquieting.

In any event, change is inevitable. The external environment is constantly evolving and thus organizations need to respond. This is particularly true with healthcare. So the challenge of leadership is to facilitate change in a positive and adaptive manner. There are many ways to accomplish this. The following outline is one individual's concept of the important principals that can aid in successfully facilitating change with a positive outcome:

- Create a Vision
- Align Your Leadership

K. C. Kent (✉)
Dean, College of Medicine, The Ohio State University, Columbus, OH, USA
e-mail: KC.Kent@osumc.edu

© Springer Nature Switzerland AG 2019
M. R. Kibbe, H. Chen (eds.), *Leadership in Surgery*, Success in Academic Surgery, https://doi.org/10.1007/978-3-030-19854-1_12

- Are You on Board?
- Create a "Burning Platform"
- Be Definitive About Your Commitment to Change
- Creating an Organizational Culture
- Lead by Example
- Speed and Timing
- Be Sensitive to Your Constituents
- A Strategy for Non-adopters
- Measure, Report and Celebrate Progress
- Be Optimistic

Create a Vision and Goals

It is essential to create and articulate a vision as well as goals for your organization, which then provides the basis for change. In most sophisticated organizations, particularly those that involve physicians, it is absolutely necessary to articulate the reason for change. Change can be particularly difficult if the reason is not clear. The vision should be simple, concise, clear, and easy to articulate. Examples might be: *our goal is to move into the top ten in NIH rankings,* or *we plan to grow our clinical volume by 20% over the next 3 years, or due to a loss of a major insurance contract we plan to reduce expenses by 10%.* There may be dozens of sub-themes that are required to accomplish each of these goals. However, the overall objective should be transparent and clear to all.

The vision should be widely distributed and repeatedly emphasized using a variety of venues. Restating the vision at meetings, through print and in conversation will lead to a widespread understanding of the overall direction of your organization. To reinforce the vision and goals, some organizations produce laminated pocket cards that provide a concise summary. For reasonably sophisticated groups this approach may be unnecessary. However, if the vision is well articulated then you should be able to solicit, at any point of time, the organization's vision and top goals from any one of your constituents. Asking an organization to change without providing a clear and logical reason will lead to failure.

Making the vision and goals aspirational, particularly the positive ones, can stimulate or excite high performing individuals. If you have the fortune of leading physicians, you are endowed with an organization of overachievers. Aspirational goals are not always met but they do push your team to reach high. That said your goals should not be unrealistic. If the target is unachievable, then no one will try. It can be frustrating to fall significantly short of one's goal, especially in an organization where the constituents are accustomed to success.

The vision or goal that you create should be logical and sensible. The loss of an important insurance contract has reduced the organizations revenue by 10%, thus the organizational budget must be diminished accordingly. Although this seems a relatively straight-forward and persuasive rationale for cutting costs, logic does not always prevail. For example, there is a common belief that under duress, organizations can manufacture money or that there are secret caches that can be called up from reserve. Another common argument made during budget reduction discussions, is that my department because of its importance to the organization, should remain budget neutral while other less important departments need to reduce expenses. All of these complexities aside, it is widely understood that all organizations need to balance their budget, thus external financial pressures make a sensible argument for internal fiscal reform. Of course, it is easier to create vision around positive rather than negative goals. Why would you not want to be top ten in the NIH rankings or who would not want to grow their clinical volume? These goals are "mom and apple pie". In a broad sense it would be almost unpatriotic to argue against these types of achievements. Regardless of whether an organization's vision and goals are positive or negative, they need to be concise, logical and reasonable in order to gain wide spread understanding and acceptance.

Align Your Leadership

With rare exception, all leaders report to an even higher level of leadership. Even a hospital CEO reports to his or her board and the Dean reports to either a board or a Chancellor. When instituting change, particularly, changes that are controversial, it is essential that your leadership be supportive. If your constituents are not satisfied with the proposed changes there is almost certainty that your leadership will become aware and or involved. Thus, it is essential that there be effective communication with your leadership before any substantial change is implemented. Leadership will feel "blindsided" if the first time they learn about a controversial decision is when they are approached by a constituent that has been negatively affected. The frequency by which you need to preemptively communicate your decisions to your leadership can vary. The most relevant factor will be the strength of your relationship and the level of trust. The question you need to ask yourself is whether your leader has confidence in your abilities. Has there been the opportunity to develop mutual trust? Will this person back you even if the decision has an unfavorable outcome? Early on in your leadership, more is better when it comes to upward communication. In addition to gaining the support of leadership for your decision, it is important to (1) gauge the strength of their support, (2) measure their individual fortitude or ability to withstand controversy and (3) assess the complexity of their and your own political environment. For controversial decisions, your leadership must be completely aligned. Moreover, they must have the strength to provide firm support regardless of the level of controversy. Lastly you need to understand the larger political environment. Your leader may not at this specific juncture, have the necessary political capital to help you implement change.

It is equally important to gain the support of key individuals other than those to whom you directly report. This would include individuals who have significant institutional influence or who are directly or peripherally affected by the proposed change. For example, if you are the Chair of Surgery, other leaders that are often affected by your decisions include other Department Chairs, the institution's Chief

Medical Officer, the Board of Trustees, other medical school or university leadership, legislators, etc. Communicating with these individuals, whether it be informational or to ask for their support, will enhance the likelihood of your initiative's success. For controversial changes, it is absolutely essential that leadership and key constituents be solidly supportive and on your team.

Are You on Board?

Passion for a change is easy to arouse if the change is part of your strategic plan. But what if you are asked to implement an organizational initiative that you do not support or is not in line with your philosophy. Or even more challenging is to implement an initiative that negatively impacts the portion of the organization that you lead. Every leader will be asked from time to time to effect changes they may not individually support. This is part of the job. There are multiple ways to accomplish the same goal and it may well be that the style or approach of your leadership differs from yours. Alternatively the initiative may negatively impact your group but be beneficial to the organization as a whole. Give and take is necessary in every leadership role; perhaps in the next negotiation the outcome will favor you. During your tenure as a leader, it is likely you will ask *your team* from time to time to implement changes that they do not personally support. Consensus is wonderful if it can be achieved, but in large organizations, forward movement requires decisive leadership. In the rare situation where the proposed change is grossly misaligned from your individual goals and principles or irreparably harmful to your team, some level of reconciliation with your leadership will be necessary. However, learning how to be accommodating and flexible is an essential part of leadership.

Create a "Burning Platform"

One of the major impediments to change is the lack of a perceived need. "It all is going well, why should we do anything differently". The lack of an imminent and compelling reason for change has led to the failure of many important initiatives. When proposing change it is worth considering whether there is a "burning platform". The concept is that the platform on which you are standing, is on fire. It will burn quickly making it imperative that you abandon the platform and move to another. The parallel for our organizations is preserving the status quo is not a viable option. It is imperative that we rapidly move to a new strategy before the organization fails. If there is an immediate, palpable and convincing need for change, the burning platform already exists. Perhaps your organization lost $50 million over the last fiscal year, or your market share is down 20% year over year. Either of these events would provide evidence that change is absolutely necessary. But often, the need for change is more subtle. Changes in health care may evolve slowly. Population health is an example of a concept that is being slowly integrating into our environment. We can choose to wait until payment models change and then be responsive, or we can change now how be prepared when the new payment models arrive. The most successful organizations are those that change proactively and prepare for the future. The task for leadership is to transform these more subtle reasons for change into a compelling "burning platform". This requires convincing your organization of the need to be proactive, and grow to the next level. The platform may be on fire but the flames are not obvious. Creating "immediacy" around a situation is a skill that all good leaders need to develop. It is the responsibility of leadership to see into the future, prepare for change and convince your organization to be proactive. Creating a burning platform is a strategy that can help convince your organization that not only is change compelling but that the time for change is now.

Be Definitive About Your Commitment to Change

For most leaders, there will come a time when your resolve will be tested. Are you truly willing or able to enforce change, particularly in the face of conflict? No one wishes to be challenged but if you are creating change, push back is inevitable. Although it is difficult to face adversity at any time during your tenure as a leader, this is particularly true early on. Nevertheless, an early challenge, if unavoidable, can also be a strategic opportunity. An early show of resolve can go a long way in sending a message to your organization about your strength as a leader and your commitment to change. Unfortunately an early show of weakness can have the counter effect. This is not to suggest that one should search for conflict. Peaceful, cooperative, and collaborative change is always the desired goal. But if this is not possible, then a show of strength is far more effective than a demonstration of weakness. There is a belief by some that conflict should be avoided at all cost during the first few months of one's leadership tenure; that difficult decisions should be made only after time has passed and political capital has been gained. The alternative view is that your political capital is greatest soon after your arrival as a new leader, and that maintenance of this capital is achieved by being consistent and firm. Regardless of the timing of change, it is critical that your constituents from the outset understand your firm and unwavering devotion to the vision and your absolute expectation that they will join in the cause.

Passion and Creating an Organizational Culture

Passion is a critical element in the process of instituting change. When trying to change culture, a leader's enthusiasm and engagement can be pivotal. When change is for the positive (i.e. growth of the organization) conveying excitement and a sense of community can engender great excitement. Even if a change is negative or disruptive, a sense of compassion and caring can go a long way in ameliorating the negative impact. Passion is one of the most important assets of any leader who is proposing change.

Along with passion it is important to articulate the reason for change in a way that resonates with the individuals who are affected. For example the goal is to encourage physicians to arrive at their clinics on time. One approach might be: "You need to be timely in clinic because the medical foundation is focused on cost and efficiency." Although this statement will resonate with leadership it may be less relevant to rank and file physicians. Alternatively the statement: "You need to be in clinic on time because your patients deserve the best and it is unfair to ask them to wait", might be received by physicians with greater enthusiasm. A capable leader is able to articulate the vision in a manner that provides a clear understanding of why this change will help achieve the core values of the organization. One of the most important attributes of a great leader is the ability to communicate and to connect on a personal level.

Many changes benefit the organization as a whole, but not specific individuals within the organization (although not always immediately obvious, if the organization benefits ultimately so do its constituents). Therein lies the need to instill in individuals an organizational culture rather than a culture of individuals. This is a difficult concept for many to grasp, particularly successful physicians. We are forced during training and early in our careers to devote significant time and energy to our own personal success. College, medical school and residency are intense experiences that require a great deal of self-absorption and focus. Consequently, it becomes challenging when we are asked, later in our careers, to leave behind the personal focus and devote time and energy to our organization or to others. One of the greatest challenges or opportunities for all leaders is build an organizational culture. How do you convince your constituents that organizational synergy can outperform the sum of individual efforts? If the organization is greatly successful and accomplished, each individual's success will be enhanced. Celebrating organizational success can be as rewarding as celebrating personal success as long as there is camaraderie and a joint mission. We can take great lessons in this regard from college sports. The best of quarterbacks becomes inconspicuous if he/she is part of a losing team, whereas even a mediocre quarterback can be successful if supported by a superb offensive line.

Lead by Example

If you as the leader provide expectations for those in your organization, it is important to impose these same expectations on yourself. If your physicians are told to arrive at clinic on time, then you should arrive 15 min early. If the goal for researchers is to have a sustainably-funded research programs, then if you conduct research, your program should also be funded. Although the adage "do as I say not as I do" may work well for parenting (it probably doesn't even work well for parenting), a "do as I say" approach is particularly ineffective for leaders. If you expect your organization to change then you should be at the front leading that change.

Speed and Timing

One of the virtues of a transformational leader is impatience, a lack of comfort with the status quo, an insatiable desire to improve and push the organization to higher levels. Many organizations have benefited from leaders with these characteristics. These traits, however, need to be balanced by a calculation of the organizations appetite for and ability to change. Moving too quickly without building consensus and allowing assimilation of the new direction can lead to failure, not only of the initiative but also of the organization's leader. There are many examples, particularly in health care, of individuals making dramatic organizational changes within the first few months of their arrival, resulting in a quick turnover of leadership. This "scorched earth" approach is rarely, albeit occasionally, effective in the world of medicine. In most circumstances, an overtly aggressive approach is not warranted or necessary.

However, there are also consequences to moving too slowly. Our external environment has no limits on how quickly it can evolve and it is necessary for leaders to keep pace. Moreover, no matter how fast you intend to move, the actual movement is always slower than you might imagine. Lastly, the organization will quickly become accustomed to your pace, whether it be a slow or fast.

The pace of change should be individualized, and will vary with the magnitude of the proposed change as well as the culture of the organization. A capable leader will be capable of weighing these factors and determining the correct pace. The middle ground is often best, however a little impatience or an edge can keep an organization awake, vibrant and progressive. One strategy is to make changes quickly but phase these changes in over time. This approach can be effective when it comes to issues of compensation. For example, the decision of an organization to reduce salaries by 10% can be challenging for its constituents. Most individuals create a lifestyle that consumes the majority of their income, thus even small reductions in salary can be consequential. However, if that reduction can be phased in over several years, this provides employees the opportunity to plan and accommodate over time. In sum, when creating change, it is necessary to balance impatience with a thoughtful calculation of the level of disruption a transformational initiative might produce. The bottom line is don't wait too long! It is rewarding as a leader if your organization in leading the way.

Be Sensitive to Your Constituents

The response to change from the members of your organization will vary dramatically. The utopia of any leader is that the entire organization will be enthusiastic and supportive of the proposed change. Of course unanimous support for any change is unusual if not remote. Constituents are usually distributed into (1) supporters, (2) those that are ambivalent, and (3) those that oppose.

The more the better, when it comes to supporters. One always needs strong allies when carrying a vision forward. Finding ways to enhance the initial size of this cohort is important.

There will be a second cohort of individuals who are ambivalent, not passionate about your vision, but not opposed. This group deserves a great deal of time, focus, and attention, as the potential of moving these individuals to the supportive cohort is much greater than persuading those who are directly opposed.

Then there will be those that will oppose your initiative. There is an obvious need to invest time and effort into this group. The first step is to learn the reasoning behind their opposition. Is it possible that that they are right and you are wrong about the proposed change? Be open-minded. Step out of the box and put yourself into their situation. What about their situation has provoked resistance? Are there work-arounds that can simultaneously achieve everyone's goals? Is there the ability to negotiate a win-win situation for these individuals and your organization? Even if you persist with your initiative, your attempt to gain insight will be recognized and will occasionally allow you to reframe your initiative in a way that is more sensible or palatable for individuals who are negatively affected by the change. Under some circumstances a compromise or a more gradual rate of change might be more beneficial than failure of the initiative or the negative impact of severe resistance. When negotiating with individuals that oppose change, it is critical to not personalize their response. It is important for leaders to understand that resistance and the anger that can follow change is most often directed to the proposed change and not to you as an individual. One of the most important lessons for all leaders is the concept of "it's just business". Those in leadership must be capable of separating their individual emotions from the strife that change brings to the people they lead.

Those that oppose change will fall into three groups: passive, passive/aggressive, or aggressive resistors. Each of these individuals poses a different set of challenges. The passive group may eventually come along although the effort involved in moving these individuals forward can be substantial. Passive/aggressive individuals will not be visibly opposed to change but will work behind the scenes to interfere. This can be a frustrating group and the most difficult to address since opposition is hidden and not overt. Aggressive individuals will be outspoken and actively campaign against change. The degree of opposition can vary from moderate to fierce. However, direct opposition is often easier to address because the issues are tangible, visible and open.

When addressing those that resist change, the approach needs to be calm, thoughtful, and most importantly respectful. Today's health care systems are evolving rapidly. Changes rarely benefit everyone. It is unusual that strategic decisions are either "right" or "wrong". It is important to have empathy. Consider the following example: A long-standing faculty member has been allowed for years to assume a moderate clinical load and perform unfunded research. As the health care environment changes, resources diminish and now this same individual must assume a full clinical load or obtain funding for their research. Little surprise that that this change would lead to resistance and unhappiness on the part of the faculty. In this person's defense, the current behavior has been tolerated, if not condoned for years. Thus, it is important, to be understanding if not empathetic to this individual's situation. A long-standing agreement is being changed. A significant investment of time, accompanied by sensitivity and a thorough explanation can be rewarding and helpful in such transitions.

A Strategy for Non-adopters

The question is how to respond when, despite your best efforts, resistance persists. There are several possible approaches. First, exceptions can be made. This strategy is usually problematic. The danger is that those who you have convinced to change, particularly individuals who were initially reluctant, will not understand why others have been excused. One has to assume that if an exception is made, the next day everyone will know. This is a strategy that should be undertaken with care; there should be a solid rationale for this approach.

If exceptions are not made, the change is substantial, and leadership stands firm, those that resist will ultimately need to be dealt with. In many circumstances this requires that they leave the organization. Often this happens organically. It becomes obvious to most reasonable individuals, if they are unwilling to accept change, that their tenure in the organization is not durable. It is rare that non-adopters, particularly those with a reasonable degree of sophistication, remain in an environment where they no longer "fit". Most of us strive to be comfortable and happy at work and we seek an environment where this is readily achievable. There are of course exceptions and some individuals will continue to be disruptive and not leave the organization. For these individuals termination will be necessary. Hopefully this is a rare occurrence. When it appears that this pathway is being considered, a preemptive conversation, suggesting the value of searching for other opportunities, can sometimes avoid the disruption and negativity that accompanies termination. When termination is necessary, the reasons should be clear and concise.

For all non-adopters, there may be a period of discussion or negotiation. During these negotiations, the leader must be thoughtful, calm, and strategic. It is critical to not play in the sandbox. Interactions need to be supportive with constant reinforcement of the positive aspects of change. E-mail interactions, particularly those that are negative, are forbidden. Recognition of each individual's viewpoints is essential. Great leaders are positive and sensitive but also unflappable and firm.

In promoting change it is critically important to remain focused on the positive; on the goals and the vision rather than the resistance. Both need tending. However, the split should be 80% positive and 20% negative. If more time and energy are devoted to the resistance, less time is available for forward movement. Many great initiatives have failed because a small group or even an individual resistor is capable of consuming all of the leader's time and attention. When under fire and in the face of significant opposition, it is sometimes difficult to focus on the positive, to embrace one's supporters, and to feel confident about the proposed change. Occasionally it is necessary to put on blinders and just continue moving forward.

Measure, Report and Celebrate Progress

Reporting or, better stated, celebrating your organization's success solidifies the commitment to change. "Our vision was to be in the top ten over the next 5 years and in our first year we have moved into top 20". We have successfully reduced our expenses by 10% yet we were able to care for more patients with higher quality. For those who have made sacrifices or who have contributed time and energy to your initiative, being congratulated and recognized for this success can be greatly rewarding. A personal or public compliment at a critical juncture can be worth more than a raise or a bonus. Be certain to celebrate your success at every possible juncture.

Be Optimistic

Never underestimate the ability of an organization or individuals in an organization to adapt and evolve. We know from Darwin that evolution sacrifices some. But humans, particularly sophisticated physicians, have an impressive ability to adapt and evolve. It is surprising how resistant individuals can be to change …maybe it actually not that surprising. But equally impressive is how capable we are of adapting, particularly if the environment is positive and supportive. There are some that readily embrace change, however, many do not. We all have the tendency to desire the status quo, particularly if it is longstanding. *But as much as individuals wish to avoid change within their organization, there is even greater resistant to changing organizations.* Usually, the lesser of two evils is to stay put and adapt. For those leaders who are adept and facilitating change, success is frequent and casualties are rare.

Conclusion

The downfall of many bright and talented leaders is their adversity to conflict or their inability to effectively manage change. Changing and organization can be exciting, innovative and actually fun, leading to a vibrant and successful enterprise. There are dozens of leadership strategies that can be employed to manage organizational change. Underlying all of these strategies should be a thoughtful and caring leader who is considerate of the organization and its people. For adaptive change, the onus is on the leader to demonstrate that the outcome of change will be beneficial to all.

Understanding Different Health Care Systems and Funds Flow Models in Surgery

Marissa C. Kuo, David O. Anderson, and Paul C. Kuo

Introduction

Academic medical centers (AMC) have historically been considered as centerpieces in the American healthcare landscape [1, 2]. Currently, however, many AMCs face financial and governance turbulence. Historically charged with delivering complex, specialized care, the AMC in the modern era is simultaneously saddled with the costs of supporting medical education and research. As the sole "safety net" provider, AMCs often treat a disproportionate share of Medicaid or under- and uninsured patients for emergency, Level 1 trauma and psychiatric crises. Increases in consumerism and competition magnify these challenges even further. Intensifying demands for price transparency combined with inconsistent and less than desirable quality ratings, and higher mortality rates, do not cast many AMCs in a favorable light. The traditional appeal and historic image of AMCs may diminish as more patients seek routine care elsewhere.

Clinical care, research, and education are recognized as the traditional pillars of academic medicine. Overlying this tripartite mission are both the structure of the academic medical center and the legal and financial ties between its traditional constituents: public or private status, for-profit or not-for-profit status, hospital (or hospitals), school of medicine (and perhaps university), faculty practice group, and affiliated community physicians. A complete discussion regarding constituents of AMCs must also consider the constantly changing financial landscape of clinical care, research and education including the various sources of revenue of each:

M. C. Kuo
Emory University School of Medicine, Atlanta, GA, USA
e-mail: mckuo@emory.edu

D. O. Anderson · P. C. Kuo (✉)
University of South Florida, Tampa, FL, USA
e-mail: doa@health.usf.edu; paulkuo@health.usf.edu

© Springer Nature Switzerland AG 2019
M. R. Kibbe, H. Chen (eds.), *Leadership in Surgery*, Success in Academic
Surgery, https://doi.org/10.1007/978-3-030-19854-1_13

Medicare, Medicaid, private insurance and its various insurance "managed care products," self-pay, philanthropy, Veterans Administration, and National Institutes of Health, among others. Governmental regulation implemented through Stark Law, Halifax decision, and inurement considerations influence overall financial strategy and inter-party negotiations attending to cost shifting, revenue sharing or gain sharing [3]. Also, trends of clinical integration, value-based healthcare, and population health further cloud the financial and regulatory framework AMCs must operate in. Understanding and navigating this ever changing, multi-tiered, jigsaw puzzle of health care delivery in the academic medical center is an ongoing challenge for all leaders in AMCs. The structure of an academic health care system and the methodology by which resources are allocated among the various entities significantly influence the conduct of the clinical, research, educational, and administrative functions of an academic department of surgery.

In the chapter that follows, we present an overview of the evolving structure of the academic medical center with examples of published funds flow models from University of Pennsylvania, Stanford University, University of California at San Francisco, and University of Alabama at Birmingham. AMCs are highly variable and individual entities. Therefore, success in achieving financial viability while simultaneously addressing the tripartite academic mission in an academic department of surgery will require ongoing vigilance, agility, fluidity, innovation and ultimately, compromise.

The Changing Structure of the Academic Health Care System

The economic engine of an academic medical center (AMC) is its clinical operation, also known as the academic health system (Fig. 13.1). The clinical enterprise represents the combined assets of the teaching hospital(s) and clinical faculty. Depending on the system, affiliated non-academic community physicians may also contribute to the clinical enterprise. Historically, the other components of the

Fig. 13.1 Structure and relationships among academic medical center components [8]

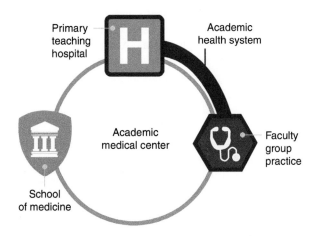

academic mission (research and teaching programs) are underfunded by their traditional revenue streams. Specifically, start-up funds required for new research programs and faculty recruitment, perpetual cost-sharing of grants, appetite for capital and technology demands are most often excluded from traditional academic revenue streams. Schools of medicine derive funding from a variety of sources including tuition, state funding, philanthropy, clinical revenues generated by the hospital and clinical faculty practice plan, and indirect money from grants. To emphasize the overall cost of research, the top 40 research intensive medical schools in the United States contributed $300 million of their own institutional funds to the operation of research centers; however, these funds are constantly being criticized and subject to reduction [4]. Despite these various sources of funding, revenue from clinical care subsidizes the research and education missions at every medical school.

Clinical care performed through hospitals, faculty practice, and other clinics generally average 85% of revenue for academic medical centers [4]. Academic medical centers may also receive additional funds through direct and indirect medical education payments. Programmatic support may also exist for services provided to the hospital which may include 24/7 physician in-house coverage, administrative roles such as medical director, IT infrastructure management, and participation in compliance and quality assurance programs. New programs for clinical growth, including recruitment of physicians, often require financial support from the hospital, often achieved through a "Professional Service or Research Support Agreement". Grants and contracts constitute the second largest single revenue source, approximately 12% of total funding. Federal grant funds are increasingly difficult to attain through national initiatives such as limits to grant support for individual PIs and efforts to consolidate federal funds into a small and finite number of research intensive organizations. All other sources combined including endowments, donor gifts, and tuition accounted for the remaining 3% [4]. The identified threats to revenues for the academic medical center include: indirect medical education funding, disproportionate share hospital payments, Medicare basket updates, state funding, new funding models including the Accountable Care Organization and bundled payments, commercial insurers creating tiered benefits and/or narrow networks, new quality standards, grant and contract funding via the NIH, philanthropy, physician sustainable growth rate, and loss of previously insured patients. This study identifies a number of strategies for the future, including but not limited to the following:

1. Building the brand by holding faculty accountable for cost and quality.
2. Becoming part of a larger community and/or regional network
3. Push the envelope on new kinds of extenders to increase effectiveness. These extenders include, technology, in addition to personnel, become an information hub to realize return on health information technology investment, align the research pipeline with clinical and business strategies [4].

The changing structures, challenges and future intentions of the academic medical center largely inform the downstream funds flow model. Clinical activity constitutes the vast majority of revenue for AMCs. As such, there are innumerable forces driving the perceived need for greater clinical integration to enhance and reinforce the clinical enterprise to be able to support the tripartite mission of the AMC:

1. Traditional academic revenue streams are declining.
2. Professional fees in faculty practice groups have declined and face additional cuts for most specialties
3. Free standing practice plans can no longer subsidize the academic mission at historical levels such as transfer vehicles such as the Dean's Tax. Pressures to recruit and retain highly productive clinical faculty require a greater amount of practice revenues and professional revenues be used to support clinical faculty compensation and clinical infrastructure.
4. Margins of major teaching hospitals are the last places for resources to fund academic mission.
5. Teaching hospital performance is a reflection of a combined effort between the clinical faculty and hospital team.

The greatest challenge facing the modern AMC is upholding its tripartite mission while simultaneously balancing the interplay of its organizational structure including the teaching hospital, medical school, and faculty practice group. Ongoing changes in the market place have rendered this challenge increasingly complex. Studies from the Association of American Medical Colleges and Institute of Medicine indicate that the success of each component is intertwined with that of each of the others [5–7]. In the face of such a challenge, many academic medical centers are making significant changes to improve their performance; as of 2015, 31% of Association of Academic Health Center members are attempting to do so by modifying their governance structures [6]. In this study, Enders and coauthors conclude that academic medical centers have four options: form a system, partner with others in a collaborative network model, merge into a system, or be prepared to shrink in isolation [6].

Modifying the governance structure of the AMC may not be sufficient to meet the growing challenges. Several studies have put forth various theories to assist in ensuring the future success of the AMC. A Price-Waterhouse study reduces the challenge at hand to three major obstacles that must be managed.

1. Budgetary and political pressures will raise the threat level at AMCs. For example, only 22% consumers surveyed by PWC said they would pay more to be treated at an academic medical center.
2. Low quality rankings and imprudent affiliations could damage the brand of the academic medical center.
3. The traditional academic medical center structures are not designed to address new challenges [4].

An additional force that necessitates the need for change for many AMCs is patient access. Same-day appointments and geographical convenience are two objectives that many AMCs have not historically considered in their deployment of resources.

A different approach outlined in a 2014 study by the Institute of Medicine examined stewardship priorities for academic health systems and identified ten qualities central to navigating the changing health care terrain in the United States [5]:

1. Enable broad engagements by families, patients and the public
2. Create and scale innovative models for efficient personal and population health management
3. Develop and leverage data, science and resources for new knowledge
4. Emphasize studies that sharply focus and pace for improved health outcomes
5. Demonstrate a continuously learning culture and practice
6. Train a well-coordinated, professional team-based work force
7. Foster an environment that develops and empowers clinical leaders
8. Forge diverse interceptor and multidisciplinary approaches
9. Help communities locally, nationally and globally access tools for better health
10. Measure and communicate the complications and impact of academic health systems.

Traditionally, the academic medical center has upheld the tripartite mission of clinical practice, research, and education. The modern-day AMC attempts to maintain this mission while simultaneously integrating the interests and goals of the teaching hospital, medical school, and faculty practice group. Innumerous threats to revenue complicate this complex and impressive goal. The current economic climate will require AMCs to make changes to their governance system, stewardship priorities, and organizational structures. Various AMCs are moving to address these concerns.

Academic Medical Center Models

Academic medical center models typically fall into one of five structures (Fig. 13.2). These include the integrated academic medical center, hospital and faculty practice aligned structure, university and faculty practice aligned structure, university and hospital alignment, and lastly, all three as separate entities. The first two represent the hospital and faculty practice group in a single structure. The last three represent structures in which the hospital and faculty practice group are independent. Although the degree of structural integration refers to the corporate governance and organization of the academic health system, the various constituents continue to have a direct vested interest in each other's success. Nevertheless, functional integration in many ways supersedes structural integration as an operational necessity.

It is generally agreed that functional integration requires enhanced coordination between the hospital and faculty practice groups within the domains of strategic planning, budgeting, capital and facilities planning, matrix reporting, clinical

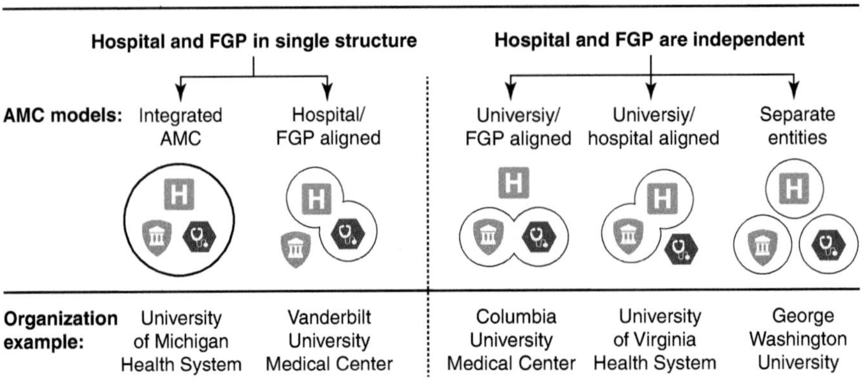

Fig. 13.2 Examples of AMC structural models [8]

service offerings, and position recruitment. Strategic planning in which goals are developed through a collaborative process reinforces the notion that entities are working toward identical goals. Collaborative development of budgets ensures synchronization. There may be contractual obligations to obtain budget approval from the other entity in certain defined situations. A multi-year capital plan developed collaboratively insures interorganizational alignment and synchronization. Joint committees may exist to evaluate decisions requiring major capital investment. Matrix reporting lines, theoretically, obligate key executives to concurrently represent and balance interests of both the academic and clinical enterprises. Typically, these positions are the Executive Vice President of Clinical Affairs, or President of the Faculty Practice Group. Decisions to add to or grow clinical services are made in a collaborative fashion. Lastly, entities may collaborate on recruitment of new physicians to fulfill long term goals of the hospital entity.

A 2015 study by ECG subdivides systems into levels of more integrated and less integrated [8] (Fig. 13.3). The more integrated systems exhibit a system-owned faculty practice group, direct physician employment, senior executive reporting relationships between the hospital and faculty practice group, university ownership of both the hospital and faculty practice group and/or the presence of a virtual/parent health system (Fig. 13.4). In contrast, less integrated system features include a school-based faculty practice plan, department-based faculty practices and/or a separate faculty practice plan and hospital. In the ECG study, they found that increased integration was associated with enhanced reputation scores, higher quality, enhanced research, improved GME functions, but decreased overall financial performance.

Keroack and co-authors examined the role of functional alignment vs. structural integrity of medical schools and teaching hospitals [9]. In their examination of 85 academic health centers, these authors found that a high degree of structural integrity was usually associated with significantly higher functional alignment, although there was considerable overlap between high and low structural integrity institutions. Notably, they found that structural integrity was not associated with enhanced performance measures, rather functional alignment was significantly associated with higher performance in teaching, research, and finance, but not clinical care and efficiency.

More integrated criteria

Characteristics	Description
System-owned FGP	The FGP is a separate legal entity but is owned or controlled by the hospital/health system.
Direct physician employment	The FGP is a business unit/division within the hospital/health system. and/or the hospital directly employs faculty/physicians.
Senior executive reporting relationships	Hospital and FGP leadership report to the same individual, and/or a hospital leader has an executive role in the FGP or vice versa.
University owned	The university owns both the hospital and the FGP. which is a separate legal entity, or the university owns the hospital, and the SOM employs the faculty of the FGP (a division of the SOM).
Virtual health system/ parent health system	There is a virtual health system (often consistent with reporting relationships), or there is a parent health system over both entities.

Less integrated criteria

Characteristics	Description
School-based FGP	The FGP is a division of the SOM with no corporate ties to the hospital. and/or the FGP is separately incorporated, but the university/SCM is the controlling entity.
Department-based FGP	Regardless of its disposition and ownership structure, the FGP has limited authority and otherwise represents or supports a department-centric organization of clinical faculty.
Separate FGP and hospital	The FGP is a separate legal entity, and regardless of its alignment with the SOM, it has no formal organizational/corporate relationship with the adult primaoy teaching hospital.

Fig. 13.3 Criteria for degrees of integration [8]

Other thought leaders have also approached the question of the structure and role of AMCs within the ever-changing landscape of healthcare. Hegwer has indicated that a number of changes would enable organizations to take on value-based payment, population health management with the rise of consumerism in healthcare [10]. These include centralizing and professionalizing the board, hiring leaders to support innovation and transformation, building and reassessing partnerships, strengthening integration, organizing physicians, retooling infrastructure to focus on quality, building a cohesive physician and ambulatory services unit, creating a value-based care and payment task force, creating alignment through organizational restructuring, and focusing on funds flow alignment. They quote Steven Klasko, President and CEO of Thomas Jefferson University and Jefferson Health, "The old math is NIH funding, inpatient revenue, and tuition for success in academic medicine. Success in the future requires new math, which focuses on academics, clinical care, innovation, and philanthropy" [10]. The structure of the academic health system, whether it evolves via structural integration or not, places a great emphasis on functional alignment. It is this functional alignment that, in turn, will determine the funds flow model for clinical departments.

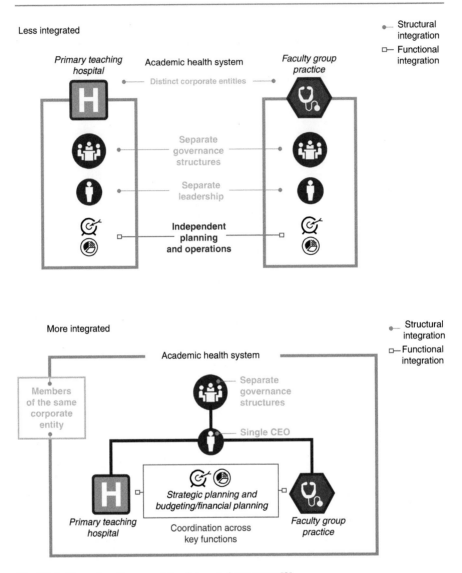

Fig. 13.4 Examples of more and less integrated structures [8]

Funds Flow

Perhaps one of the greatest misconceptions endured by both academic physicians and leadership of AMCs is the perceived variability and inconsistency in the understandings of the source of funds and use of funds in AMCs. The grass always seems to be greener and highly skilled professionals frequently discuss and analyze this topic at varies forums such as professional meetings, conferences, etc. At the macro and highest level of an AMC, the methodology and mechanics of receiving funds and expending funds is extremely consistent. There is a finite way funds can be received and spent. The confusion and need for clarity and communication begins once the funds are internally distributed at the micro level of an AMC. Nevertheless, transparency, alignment, and effective communication of the internal or micro funds flow is the mechanism to resolve organizational barriers to drive future viability and survival.

Funds flow insures alignment, drives accountability, supports enterprise level goals and financial sustainability, reinforces excellence in academic missions, and preserves flexibility to adapt to changing needs. For funds flow to be effective, the methodology for funding must be transparent, rational, trusted and mutually accepted by physician leaders. The future success of the academic medical center will rely on appropriate and high yield resource allocation. It is critical that every academic medical center establish a structured and disciplined approach for funding the three missions of the enterprise. This approach may be broken down into four stages: 1) Analyzing the cash inflows and outflows so all stakeholders understand both macro and micro fund flows of an AMC 2) Rationalizing and simplifying the existing flow of funds, 3) Defining a transparent and role- driven model, that is consistent across time and 4) Laying the groundwork for sustainability through process, policy, governance and controls. Data must be normalized by creating a common data model and then mapped to the existing accounts. Key performance indicators for each funding category should be defined and linked to funding provided, in order to measure effectiveness and drive accountability.

A critical component of funds flow centers on a transparent, simple, and equitable methodology for clinical faculty compensation and productivity. These are typically benchmarked using one or more of the following market surveys: 1) AAMC Medical School Faculty Salary Survey, 2) UHC-AAMC Faculty Practice Solutions Centers Productivity Data, 3) AMGA Medical Group Compensation and Financial Survey, 4) MGMA Physician Compensation and Production Survey, 5) Sullivan Cotter Large Clinic Physician Compensation Survey and/or Sullivan Cotter Physician Productivity Survey Report. There is considerable variability amongst academic medical centers as to which market survey is used. Nevertheless, consistency and transparency of survey selection and utilization is of paramount importance for faculty buy-in and confidence.

University of Pennsylvania Model

In a description of the University of Pennsylvania model, Kennedy and co-authors describe the approach to their funds flow reallocation process that took place in 2004 [11]. The process was based on the following principles: 1) align with the overall Penn Medicine strategic plan, 2) be fair and transparent, 3) match revenue with expenses based on a rational value-based model, 4) provide appropriate incentives to be put in place to encourage achieving and/or exceeding system growth objectives, 5) individual faculty clinical activity expectations were established, tied a compensation schema and communicated, at least annually, 6) funds flow should provide for opportunity for gain sharing related to future margin growth, and 7) measure and monitor over time. As an example of the various categories of the clinical components of funds flow, the authors describe new program start up in 1) recruitment, 2) purchased services by faculty for administrative regulatory or directorship activities, 3) programmatic support which may be exemplified by support from the hospital for clinical programs which the health system deems important and the practices lose money, 4) incentive payment for gain sharing around financial improvement and 5) pass through and payer contracts in which third party contract payments encompassing global payments to the system are then allocated to hospital and physician practices. In order to maintain chair flexibility and autonomy, the majority of funds were allocated at the department level. Following implementation of this new funds flow model, the authors note that total funding for clinical departments increased 30.8% between FY05 ($121M) and FY07 ($159M), while the school of medicine contribution of the total decreased by 25% to $9M during this time. The largest proportion of the increase was associated with new hires, support for clinical program strategic growth, inflationary increases in teaching, research, and clinical purchased services, academic development funds, and enhanced third-party pass through resulting from additional volume on global contracts. The authors conclude that the integrated nature of the Penn health system and the new funds flow methodology were significant factors in their financial improvement. They recommend that a broad evaluation such as that performed at Penn might benefit other AMCs.

Stanford University Model

The Stanford University funds flow model encompasses hospitals which are separate 501(c)(3)s owned by the University, operate all clinical facilities (inpatient, outpatient and ancillaries), assume risk and reward for the clinical enterprise (including, payor mix), and perform all contracting, billing and collections and are responsible for malpractice [12, 13]. The adult funds flow 5-year agreement was originally established in 2006 and renegotiated in 2011 and 2016. The objectives were intended to:

1. Align outcomes and incentives between the Stanford Hospital and Clinics and the School of Medicine
2. Be simple, formula-driven, stable, predictable and transparent
3. Include the full range of professional services and funding, such as clinical services, medical administrative services, program development and mission-based funding
4. Support increased productivity and market-based compensation for physicians
5. Incentivize physicians to enhance the clinical enterprise and ensure high quality care and service standards.

The broad outline of the Stanford funds flow model includes WRVU payments for physician clinical work based on median MGMA total compensation per WRVU and by specialty. In addition, there are department transfers for physician benefits, clinical department overhead costs, Dean and University taxes on clinical revenue, GME program director costs, medical director costs, program development support for new recruits, quality, safety and service initiatives and academic grants, including the share to the Dean's office. Following implementation of this funds flow model, WRVU payments were increased from the MGMA 50th to the MGMA 75th percentile and the shared margin trigger decreased from 6.5% to 4%. Finally, quality safety and services incentives were increased to 8% from 6% of WRVUs.

University of California—San Francisco (UCSF) Model

In 2014, at UCSF the rapid increase in cost of practice over the increase in professional fee revenues began rendering many clinics financially unsustainable. As a result, UCSF administration realized the need for a new funds flow model between the Medical Center and School Of Medicine [14, 15]. The previous model was based on professional revenue as the source of payment for clinical expenses associated with physician practices. Departments managed all practice and departmental clinical and faculty expenses independently and clinical income was supplemented by hundreds of individual agreements between the Health System and departments. The numerous, complex strategic support agreements had become unwieldy, difficult to adequately communicate, and increasingly expensive. Patients' experience was highly variable from one clinic to the next. The existing clinical funds flow model was complex, non-transparent, growth-inhibiting, access-limiting, and financially unsustainable.

The aim of the new funds flow design was for all individuals who spent the majority of their time supporting the clinical enterprise to be housed under a single organizational structure. The goals were defined as: clinical growth, financial sustainability, academic mission, efficiency, enhanced patient access, competitive compensation, and long-term viability. The UCSF Health System was defined as all components of the clinical organization, including the UCSF Medical Center and the Physician Practices. The Health System would collect the professional and technical revenue for clinical services and be responsible for all patient care expenses, including practice, clinical department, and faculty productivity expenses. Departments were given the responsibility for faculty salaries and any remaining departmental expenses. Practice decisions were made collaboratively between the Health System and each department and individual agreements between the Health System and the departments were limited. Professional fees and technical revenue accrued to the Health System. The Health System assumed financial responsibility for the cost of operating ambulatory and inpatient practices with the exception of the cost of physician and faculty clinical effort. Four tiers of payment to the departments' clinical income stream were established:

1. A dollar per WRVU payment made to the department for various subspecialties determined using national standards for physician productivity and compensation.

2. Margin sharing incentive payment in which the health system, clinical departments, and Dean's office share in a margin earned above the annual combined budget for the health system.
3. An incentive plan to align the health system and departments' goals designed to enhance quality, access, and patient experience.
4. A staffing payment reserved for a small number of clinical services for which physician staffing is a requirement for safety, regulatory mandates or mission critical for patient care.

In addition, the Health System reimbursed the departments for actual benefits expense related to faculty clinical time and pay for clinical operating overhead expense. Finally, the health system paid the malpractice expenses, absorbed all expenses associated with billing and coding, Dean's tax, all medical group expenses, and much of the expense related to ambulatory practices.

University of Alabama (UAB) Model

At UAB, the leadership found that existing hospital mission support processes did not align the faculty practice with the hospital practice [16]. Departments were requesting more funds than were needed and selected departments were experiencing financial difficulty despite receiving mission support. Multiple specialties performing the same procedures were receiving different conversion rates. The rational underlying the change to funds flow included healthcare reform, changing reimbursement models, and insuring the survival of the UAB Health System clinical and academic missions. Anticipated outcomes included organizational leadership alignment across the academic medical center, transparency of finances at both the departmental and divisional level, alignment of incentives, and clinical integrational of quality outcomes.

The new UAB funds flow model eliminated all previous hospital support and centralized all clinical costs. Compensation was based upon WRVUs; WRVU revenues were based upon a 3-year rolling average based on the average MGMA compensation per WRVU. The salary goal was 70% of median MGMA by specialty. Within the Dept. of Surgery, there were ten divisions and 21 resulting rates of WRVU revenues. At non-UAB hospitals, such as the Children's Hospital of Birmingham, professional fees and clinical expenses remained in place and physician benefit and departmental administrative cost reimbursement were maintained. There was a withhold established at 10% of RVU revenues linked to 20 at risk metrics created to enable return. These metrics were based on a combination of practice performance metrics, including patient satisfaction, quality and finance. Individual departments developed WRVU-based compensation plans encompassing their academic, clinical, and educational missions.

A shared governance structure, consisting of a cooperative effort between the faculty practice and the hospital, implemented the new model which removed infrastructure and clinical expense from departmental responsibility, thus enhancing the financial performance of many clinical departments. Furthermore, the new model permitted the implementation of an academic enrichment fund to the School of Medicine. Subsequent years found that the combined performance of the hospital and practice plan in FY15 was significantly favorable to budget with a variance of $69 million with respect to FY14. The Dept. of Surgery experienced a $6.1 million and $5.1 million operating margin in FY14 and FY15, respectively and FY15 total WRVUs was >885,000. A retrospective review of the prior funds flow model concluded the new funds flow model improved the clinical operating margin and reserves of various departments, many of which were able to receive WRVU revenues regardless of the payor mix, and Dept. Chairs were empowered to distribute revenue for recruitment, retention, and the academic mission.

Conclusion

"A revolution under way in health care is fundamentally changing how every academic medical center operates" [6]. AMCs are reexamining relationships and funding priorities. Functional integration is underway to leverage both professional and hospital revenue to not only support and sustain the traditional missions of clinical care, research, and education, but also more fundamentally, to ensure the future viability of the AMC. For an academic dept. of surgery within this AMC, the funds flow model design determines future investment and apportionment among the various missions.

In the future, not all AMC's will achieve equal success. Particularly vulnerable are the education and research missions. Top performing AMCs will quickly streamline and effectively execute both strategy and operations based upon a common definition and understanding of both macro and micro fund flows of the organization. Resource allocation and performance metrics will require stakeholders and decision-makers to be more agile and responsive to outcome data. Even though there are several structural models that may exist, execution, alignment and communication will dictate success.

References

1. McCue MJ, Thompson JM. Analysis of cash flow in academic medical centers in the United States. Acad Med. 2011;86(9):1100–7.
2. Itri JN, Mithqal A, Krishnaraj A. Funds flow in the era of value-based health care. J Am Coll Radiol. 2017;14(6):818–24.
3. Bulleit T, Caron MM, Peloquin D. New frontiers in AMC funding: mission support alternatives post halifax; 2017. Accessed on 23 Aug 2018. Available from: https://www.healthlawyers.org/Members/PracticeGroups/Documents/AMC-TH_Topical_Library/Program_Paper_bulleit_wahler.pdf.
4. Barnes K, Valletta R. The future of the Academic Medical Center: PwC Health Research Institute; 2012. Available from: http://www.aahcdc.org/Portals/41/AIM-Program/Best-Practices/Financial_Alignment/The_Future_of_the_Academic_Medical_Center_Strategies_to_Avoid_Margin_Meltdown.pdf.

5. Dzau VJ, Gottlieb G, Lipstein S, Schlichting N, Washington E. Essential stewardship priorities for academic health systems. NAM perspectives [Internet]; 2014. Available from: https://nam.edu/wp-content/uploads/2015/06/AcademicHealthSystems.pdf.

6. Enders TC, Conroy J. Advancing the academic health system for the future: Association of Academic Medical Colleges; 2014. Available from: https://www.aamc.org/initiatives/patient-care/aphc/357864/academichealthsystem.html.

7. Mann S. New report encourages leaders to envision the future of academic medicine. AAMC news [Internet]; 2016. Accessed on 23 Aug 2018. Available from: https://news.aamc.org/research/article/faculty-engagement-advancement/.

8. Collins C, Horrison D, Potter K, Banty K. Are integrated academic health systems better?; 2015. Accessed on 23 Aug 2018. Available from: http://www.ecgmc.com/thought-leadership/whitepapers/are-integrated-academic-health-systems-better.

9. Keroack MA, McConkie NR, Johnson EK, Epting GJ, Thompson IM, Sanfilippo F. Functional alignment, not structural integration, of medical schools and teaching hospitals is associated with high performance in academic health centers. Am J Surg. 2011;202(2):119–26.

10. Hegwer LR. New structures new roles for the future of health care; 2016. Accessed on 23 Aug 2018. Available from: http://www.hfma.org/Leadership/Archives/2016/Spring/New_Structures,_New_Roles_for_the_Future_of_Health_Care/.

11. Kennedy DW, Johnston E, Arnold E. Aligning academic and clinical missions through an integrated funds-flow allocation process. Acad Med. 2007;82(12):1172–7.

12. Cohen M, Comstock M, Day T, Meeks C. Funds flow models – budget consistency in academic medical centers; 2015. Accessed on 23 Aug 2018. Available from: https://s36.a2zinc.net/clients/mgma/MGMA15/Custom/Handout/Speaker0_Session897_1.pdf.

13. Stanford Health Care & Stanford University School of Medicine. Stanford clinical funds flow model; 2016. Accessed on 23 Aug 2018. Available from: https://www.yumpu.com/en/document/view/17892310/funds-flow-model-stanford-university-school-of-medicine.

14. UCSF. New clinical funds flow overview; 2014. Available from: https://fundsflow.ucsf.edu/new-clinical-funds-flow-overview.

15. UCSF. Funds flow overview: manager's meeting; 2014. Accessed on 23 Aug 2018. Available from: https://fundsflow.ucsf.edu/sites/fundsflow.ucsf.edu/files/Funds%20Flow%20Overview_Manager%27s%20Meeting_09-23-14.pdf.

16. Bland KI. University of Alabama Birmingham funds flow model; 2015. Accessed on 23 Aug 2018. Available from: https://www.facs.org/~/media/.../outcomes%20at%20uab%20%20kirby%20bland.ashx.

Understanding Different Compensation Models in Surgery

14

Bryan Clary

Overview

While it would be obvious that surgical compensation plans are of great importance to faculty, it is important for surgical leaders to recognize that there are additional key stakeholders including their institutions, trainees, and most importantly their patients. The latter may not be cognizant of the specifics of the compensation structure of their surgeons, but they are no less affected by the behaviors that may arise as a consequence of the direct and indirect incentives inherent in the plans. Trainees in the environment likewise are also potentially impacted by the ways in which faculty are compensated for clinical and educational activities.

The development of compensation plans for surgical faculty is amongst the most difficult and challenging aspects of surgical leadership. The balance of fairness, financial stewardship, and mission alignment can be tricky and the conversations with faculty can be amongst the more contentious and awkward that leaders will experience. There is a very human element to compensation plans that must be recognized and valued by surgical leaders whose faculty often carry substantial debt associated with their education and who are subject to the delayed nature of asset accumulation inherent in protracted surgical training. Compensation plans are interpreted (justly so) by faculty to reflect the priorities of their leaders. Furthermore, they conflate compensation levels with absolute levels of "worth" as perceived by their leaders and organization which has important implications on their overall job satisfaction. Given these and other considerations, compensation plans are a primary tool by which surgical leaders can affect the culture and performance of their units and operationally achieve their goals. Ill-conceived or poorly executed compensation plans are a direct pathway for failure in leadership.

B. Clary (✉)
Department of Surgery, UC San Diego Health, San Diego, CA, USA
e-mail: bclary@ucsd.edu

© Springer Nature Switzerland AG 2019
M. R. Kibbe, H. Chen (eds.), *Leadership in Surgery*, Success in Academic
Surgery, https://doi.org/10.1007/978-3-030-19854-1_14

Almost all compensation plans are local in their structure reflecting variations in professional reimbursement rates, regional competition for surgeons, institutional financial health, health system financial support models, academic expectations, and the nuances of leadership. The leadership level at which compensation plans are decided upon are also variable (i.e. health system or practice plan, department, divisional) such that in some instances surgical leaders may not directly determine the structure of the plan. Even in such circumstances, there are typically opportunities for surgical leadership to affect the structure of these plans and certainly the execution of, and impact upon their faculty. Understanding your faculty and the local environment as well as who you are competing against for talented faculty is thus critical for surgical leaders who are faced with constructing and implementing optimal compensation plans. This chapter seeks to address fundamental issues in the construction and execution of surgical compensation plans as a means of facilitating the success of surgical leaders. It is no doubt incomplete and cannot provide an exact blueprint for each compensation plan. The ideas and themes though should be of great assistance to leaders as they set about the very important task of implementing plans that are optimal for their environments.

Role of the Compensation Plan

A common misperception of compensation plans is that their principal purpose is to provide fair compensation for faculty. While this is a critical and necessary feature, the principal role of a compensation plan is to facilitate the successful execution of the unit's missions set before them by institutional leadership. Stated differently, the compensation plan must be in alignment with the goals and needs of the parent organization (practice group or health system). It must foster and facilitate optimal care for patients in a way that is financially tenable. In academic environments, the plans must also facilitate the execution of effective educational programs, sustainable and relevant research, and professional development of faculty. It is critical not only for surgical leaders to understand this basic tenant, but for them to effectively deliver this message to their faculty.

When considering salary plans it is important to recognize that there are many non-salary elements through which faculty are valued and/or are remunerated. For many faculty, these non-salary elements may be quite substantial and very important and may offset modest unmet salary expectations.

- Intrinsic satisfaction with excelling at challenging tasks
- Patient appreciation and/or achieving excellent results for patients
- Benefits (insurance, retirement, etc.)
- Resources that facilitate success in areas important to them
  - Clinical support (trainees, etc.)
  - Research support (pilot grants, research staff, travel funds, etc.)
- Professional development
  - Academic promotions

- Development of niche/content expertise
- Professional society engagement
- Participation in the affairs of the unit and overall organization
- Visible and substantive acts of appreciation by surgical leadership

It is generally unwise and inappropriate to rely on these and other non-salary elements to cover up for insufficient levels of compensation or unfair plan structures. Nonetheless, attention to these elements is important for overall faculty satisfaction and may facilitate alignment of faculty with the salary decisions of surgical leaders which they will often disagree with. For academic institutions, benefit levels (retirement, insurance, etc.) are often substantially better than those offered in private practice environments and can be quite useful to attracting candidates to situations where salary compensation may be less.

Desirable Characteristics of Compensation Plans

It has been said that "if you have seen ten different surgical compensation plans, then you have seen ten different compensation plans," a point emphasizing how heterogeneous such plans can be. While much of the heterogeneity is explained by local factors, it would also be safe to assume that there are no perfect plans. Well-performing plans do share a number of features though.

- Faculty can easily understand the structure and process
- Attractive in their ability to recruit and retain faculty
- Financially viable for the organization (departments, health system, etc.)
- Seek to minimize behaviors that are not in alignment with optimal patient care
- Fair and non-discriminatory

Faculty compensation plans that are complex and difficult to understand suffer in their implementation as faculty are not certain as to how to respond. Additionally, most faculty value clarity and want to be engaged. An opaque compensation structure precludes them from doing so and engenders feelings of distrust. Leaders must be cognizant of the physician market surrounding them. This is often difficult as the levels of compensation in competing institutions are not always readily available. Benchmark analyses (MGMA, AAMC, Sullivan-Cotter, etc.) suffer from a number of problems including over-generalization of specialized phenotypes, modest numbers of practices included in the analyses, and an imperfect appreciation of local factors including cost of living, malpractice, etc. Faculty will often relay verbally or via an offer draft sheet the terms at competing employers and while these can be useful, they must be taken at face value. The premiums demanded by new recruitments and critical retentions can create very significant imbalances internally that must be carefully considered both for financial viability of the unit and for the internal disparities they might create.

The issue of fairness within compensation plans is quite complex. There are many challenges in creating "fair" and non-discriminatory compensation plans. Firstly, leaders and faculty will often disagree on what is "fair". For example, should the plan factor in seniority (i.e. higher base salary for older faculty) irrespective of productivity metrics? Should clinical incentives be capped to facilitate a more even distribution of clinical work despite differences amongst the faculty in clinical ability and work ethic (is this fair to patients as well as faculty?). Should new recruits and or retentions merit salary premiums? Should division leaders be paid an administrative stipend through faculty taxes to support their salaries? How does the plan accommodate leaves related to illness and the birth of children?

Another challenge in the creation of "fair" plans lies in the fact that faculty even within specialty groups often have very different phenotypes with respect to clinical sub-specialization and the other activities. The various activities of faculty (clinical, administration, education, research, and others) are associated with differential levels of salary revenue generation and can thus lead to differences in compensation without strategic interventions. In an academic environment the lower revenue generating activities are critical and must be carried out. Identifying appropriate strategies for compensation of these efforts is one of the more difficult tasks that surgical leaders have to face. In the current era, most leaders would aspire to the ethos of "equal pay for equal work". While this is a great slogan and worthwhile objective, implementation is not always straightforward. One principal reason is that the opportunity to produce "equal work" is not present in many environments. Faculty do not always have complete control over their practices, their revenues, and their expenses. Systemic imbalances in health system support (i.e. medical directorships, strategic support, call-coverage payments, etc.) and referral opportunities complicate this.

Compensation Plan Governance

There are a number of models for the governance of surgical compensation plans. These can be simplified into the following major categories:

- Health system or Medical Group leadership (benchmark driven policy, rate-setting committees)
- Departmental/Division Leadership with minimal faculty engagement (Chair/Division Chief/Vice-Chair Finance)
- Departmental/Division with robust faculty engagement (departmental compensation committee)

The ability for you as a leader to influence the compensation plan depends greatly on the governance model at your institution. For leaders working within the Veterans Affairs hospitals for example, the compensation levels are set system-wide thus precluding your ability to heavily influence the process. In the traditional non-integrated (where there is a relative independent faculty practice group) academic medical center model, compensation plans are constructed at the Department level working within the construct of their faculty practice groups. In many integrated academic medical centers, the compensation plans often require assent of the health system's governing body or perhaps the faculty medical group governing body. Even in these settings though the plans are typically department-led and as such subject to significant influence by surgical leadership. When plans are Department based, there are a number of governance decisions that have to be made. Specifically, who within the Department creates and approves the plans. In some departments, the plan is largely decided upon by the Chair in collaboration with a small leadership group (Division chief, departmental business manager, Vice-Chair of finance). An alternative to this that is present in a number of departments is to utilize a faculty committee with broader representation including from different ranks, specialties, and phenotypes. There are important implications to leaders with respect to which model is present. In environments where you as a leader are able to heavily influence the plan, you can incorporate your values and priorities. The plan will be seen by your charges as reflective of your priorities and the culture you intend to preside over in the department. Even when salary models are established outside of one's level of influence, surgical leaders must still be invested in managing the consequent behaviors that arise in response the structure of the plan. Ultimately it is your responsibility as a faculty leader to ensure that the compensation plan serves to accomplish the goals of the institution and your surgical unit.

Thoughts on Incentives

One common conundrum that the leaders of compensation plans face is what the proper roles of incentives and penalties should be. The scope of this chapter is not sufficient to render a proper and thorough treatment of the scientific underpinnings of motivation, but there are a few important points that are worth considering. Firstly, assigning a dollar amount (directly or indirectly via work-RVU assignments) to a specific activity (e.g. authoring a publication, giving lecture, taking call, serving on medical center committees, etc.) will in effect be interpreted as assigning value. Such an effort whether intentional or not, will send a signal of how you as the leader value different activities. In addition, providing low or modest salary support for specific activities may "commoditize" these activities whereby they are seen as lower quality elective contributions that perhaps are not worth pursuing or taking on. There are a number of strategies one can take to engage surgical faculty in the basic activities of the group. The first and foremost of these is to lead by example. As a leader it is critical for your groups to see you as fully engaged and equally invested in the seemingly mundane or lower revenue generating activities of the department. In your participation as a leader, faculty must not perceive that you are being rewarded differentially for these activities (i.e. they are separate from your higher-level administrative functions). Secondly, surgical leaders must work with their groups to establish what it means to be a faculty member and specifically what the baseline expectations are and what the benefits to them are in belonging to the environment. Lastly, it is important to define "above and beyond" activities that are facilitated by appropriate salary support. For example, while teaching in the clinics and operating room is part of the baseline expectations for faculty functioning in academic medical centers, there are other educational roles (residency program director, medical student clerkship director, vice-chair of education) that require salary support in order to carve out the extra time required to fulfill the role. Some leaders argue for the creation of an RVU system for most of the educational and academic activities occurring within the environment. This can be cumbersome and risks devaluing or commoditizing important and necessary functions as discussed above.

Many compensation plans incorporate incentives directed at clinical volume, efficient expense management (profitability), quality metrics, and academic achievements. Properly constructed incentives will be perceived as a reward for performance above baseline expectations. Improperly constructed "incentives" are perceived as part of the expected baseline pay and when not received by faculty generate a significant amount of discord. It is important to note that surgeons are similar to the general population in that their decisions when faced with economic judgements do not always follow rationale lines of thinking. This is in accordance with the Nobel Prize winning work of Daniel Kahneman (Awardee 2002 in Economic Sciences) and Amos Traversky who developed the framework (Prospect Theory) to understand seemingly irrational behavior of individuals when faced with what appears to be identical alternative options. Prospect theory holds that people generally value gains and losses differently and will make decisions on perceived gains rather than on perceived losses. For that reason, a person faced with two equal choices that are presented differently (one in terms of possible gains and one in terms of possible losses) is likely to choose the one suggesting gains, even if the two choices yield the same end result. For example, individuals find more joy in finding $50 on the street than they would by losing $50 and subsequently finding a $100 dollar bill despite the fact that the net value of the outcomes is identical. The implications of this with respect to compensation plans is found in the practice of "holdbacks" that are embedded in compensation plans. A "holdback" refers to a set amount or percentage of compensation that is released only after a faculty member reaches a specific productivity or profitability metric. For example, a holdback approach would assign an expected salary of $300,000 with a 10% holdback ($30,000) whereby only $270,000 would be distributed unless the faculty member meets a delineated productivity target. This would be in contrast to assigning an expected salary of $270,000 with incentive opportunities of $30k for reaching the same target. Prospect theory would predict that despite the same financial outcome, that faculty would be more distressed by the former and more likely to respond to the latter in a favorable and productive manner. This is counterintuitive to some leaders who approach the increased sensitivity faculty may have with "holdbacks" as a valuable tool in driving faculty to achieve certain levels of performance. Given the importance of faculty satisfaction in the overall performance of surgical units (aside from issues of empathy and compassion), the avoidance of negative elements in the compensation plan would be generally viewed as desirable, especially when the same or better result can be obtained through more positive strategies.

There are a number of additional important decision points when incorporating incentives into the compensation plan. Firstly, what are the eligibility criteria to participate in the incentive program (i.e. are the "good citizenship" criteria, are part-time employees eligible, etc.). Are incentives to be individual or team-based? What are the specific activities to be covered under the incentives and how should productivity target levels for these activities be determined? Should incentive opportunities be capped? What percentage of expected total compensation levels should be delivered in base and incentive pay respectively? A corollary question is what to do with revenues that are generated from these activities but not paid out because faculty do not reach specified performance targets. General principles would dictate that the incentive program in the compensation plans are financially viable for the unit, are transparent and understood by faculty, are in alignment with the missions of the institution and goals of leadership, and importantly address activities that are under the control of the faculty. Optimal incentive plans in my view should compromise only a modest amount of faculty total compensation. Limits on individual clinical productivity incentives can be useful facilitating a broader distribution of work. For example, individual uncapped incentives on clinical activity may lead to hoarding of patients by faculty with well developed practices and thus interfere with the development and financial security of junior faculty. Team based incentives are particularly important in groups that employ team coverage models such as trauma/critical care, emergency medicine, and transplantation. Team-based clinical productivity targets can also be useful in groups where practices are largely individualized as they tend to foster collaborative and collective behaviors.

Revenue Sources for Compensation Plans

The pool of resources to support faculty compensation is relatively limited, but need to be understood by surgical leaders who are tasked with developing and implementing compensation plans. These sources include the following:

- Professional fees from clinical activities
- Collections (contractual, cash)
  - Fee for service
  - Capitated payments from at-risk contracts
- Funds flow care payments
- Purchased Services
- Call coverage
- Directorships
- External contracts
- Research grant salary support
- Direct employment model (VA Affairs, etc.)
- Health System incentives and/or strategic support
- Faculty start-up investments
- Other strategic support to enable market based compensation levels

- Philanthropy/Endowed Professorships
- Governmental (State) funds to support teaching/research
- Research Indirect Cost Recovery (variable policies at different institutions)

It is critical for surgical leaders to understand the nuances of these different sources including how they flow through the health system to faculty members and whether they are assessed along the way (taxed or net less expenses attributed to the faculty member). A lengthier conversation of the flow of funds within the health system is to be found in Chap. 13. For clinically active faculty, the overwhelming majority of salary supporting revenue is associated with clinical activities in the form of direct collections procured by the billing and revenue team in their medical group net of medical group expenses, institutional taxes, and departmental clinical expenses attributed to their faculty. Included in this bucket are fee-for-service work-RVU (wRVU) associated collections and the share of capitated contracts. In most academic environments surgical leaders through their power to tax these revenues may redistribute dollars from one faculty member to another. In integrated health systems that employ a funds flow model, clinical activity revenues are in the form of care payments to the departments which in most models are pegged at a specialty benchmark dollar per wRVU level. Faculty may also receive salary supporting revenues from the hospital/health system via purchase service agreements for non-wRVU generating activities such as taking call and performing administrative duties (directorships). These payments are subject to fair market value assessments which incorporate effort reporting (time) and local physician market compensation levels.

Faculty may also perform duties covered by external clinical and research purchased service agreements. This includes research salary support from the NIH, Department of Defense, private foundations, and industry among others. In some instances, these dollars flow through the Department to the faculty member whereas in others (such as the VA Affairs), faculty are paid directly without the flow of funds through the Department. There is typically a substantial gap between the average surgeon salary levels and most non-clinical purchased service salary revenues requiring the Department to find alternative revenue streams for supplementation. For example, the NIH maximum salary for awards issued after January 7, 2018 is $189,600. Educational support from institutional GME for program leadership are equally limited as are medical directorships from the hospital and clinics. Surgical leaders face enormous challenges in finding alternative funding streams to pay research and educational faculty competitive surgeon salaries with such limitations. Endowed professorships, other philanthropic support, and redistribution of clinical revenues from other faculty are the principal mechanisms available to leaders to achieve this. Most leaders would not see the goal as eliminating the entire differential between clinical care salary revenues and academic salary for both practical reasons and in the context of ensuring that the clinical programs are optimally functioning. As such, expectations and the inherent motivations of those faculty who are engaged in academic support activities are fundamental to optimizing the compensation levels and overall faculty satisfaction. It is worth noting that faculty employed within academia are in general, accepting of *modest* compensation differentials relative to those engaged primarily in non-academic private practice.

Hospitals and health systems may also support faculty salary levels through strategic support directed through the departments. Examples include time-limited startup funding for new hires who will take time to develop clinical practices and hence clinical salary supporting revenues. Health systems also can direct strategic investment dollars to the department to cover competitive salary for needed, yet underfunded established faculty ("loss leaders"). At the end of the day, the leaders of the surgical compensation plan need to tally up the expected revenues that are available for compensation and develop conservative and fair distribution plans. If there are inadequate resources, then a plan of advocacy with health system leadership as well as strategic plans to increase the pool of dollars must be generated.

Basic Models for Compensation

The time-honored basic models for compensation include (A) Individual P&L Driven Compensation and (B) Fixed Salary (Fig. 14.1). Most plans are a hybrid of the two, but it is instructive to review both.

The "Individual P&L" plan is commonly referred to as "Eat What You Kill" although in our profession most find that term objectional for many reasons. In this model the faculty member receives in total compensation the net of their attributed revenues less their expenses. How often the revenues and expenses are reconciled varies among practices and institutions. Most plans of this type incorporate a defined base salary that is based on prior year receipts and that also incorporates a baseline academic salary for being a faculty member (typically a small component of salary). There are important nuances in defining what are attributable expenses and the degree of control that faculty have over these. Expenses include institutional taxes, department/divisional taxes, medical group level expenses, and individual level expenses (personal executive assistant, travel, association dues, etc.). Faculty on an individual level often have little control over the medical group billing efficiency as

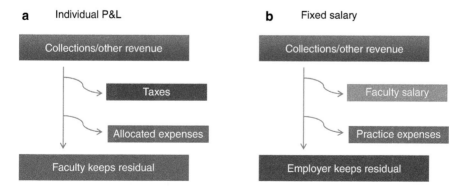

Fig. 14.1 Basic models of faculty compensation

well as complex medical group expenses that are often difficult to separate out by individual faculty members. Proponents of this approach would argue that it pushes control of expenses to the end user where the most control perhaps exists and that it is the most powerful way to increase clinical volumes given the direct and robust linkage between clinical activity and individual faculty remuneration. Given the primacy of clinical revenue in the surgical units (and hospital) and its importance in subsidizing academic activities, leaders who prefer this model see it as helpful to the overall performance of the unit. There are important downsides though. Firstly, there is an inherent perverse incentive to overtreat patients such that very careful oversight of utilization is required in such plans. Unequal and perhaps suboptimal distribution of patients amongst the group members and challenges in cross-coverage and rounding are often present as are inequalities in the distribution of resources needed to maintain and develop practices (residents, mid-level providers, etc.). An inappropriate emphasis on payor mix is also a risk whereby providers may be discouraged from taking care of underinsured patients. This model also discourages non-billable (rounding, care utilization meetings, etc.) and non-clinical activities which can lead to shortages in the coverage of these activities. One of the underlying challenges in the current era with this model when outside of an integrated health system funds flow model is that incoming revenues may be inadequate to cover allocated expenses and competitive salaries.

A fixed salary model on the other hand guarantees a faculty member a set level of compensation irrespective of volume and profitability. Excess collections/receipts if there are any are kept by the unit. In some academic departments the excess revenue is kept centrally at the department level and in others it remains within the division or section. Fixed salary models are most common in integrated health systems where the surgical units function in a zero-budget environment (i.e. where the accumulation of reserves are precluded and where subsidization of non-clinical missions is minimal). Salaries at the entry level are often quite competitive with private practice and academia. The ability to generate higher salaries through individual and/or group productivity is muted though such that more clinically active and senior surgeons draw higher salaries in the private practice and academic environments. Examples of fixed salary models are found in the Veterans Affairs Hospitals, active military, HMO's, and a few academic programs. It is worth noting that modest bonus opportunities may exist in these environments although they are not typically related to clinical volumes, but instead to patient care metrics. Proponents of fixed compensation models feel that the lack of linkage to the volume of clinical activity provides a more regular and controllable working environment that is best at avoiding unnecessary medical care. The HMO's employing these models are commonly the lowest cost health systems in the market that present more affordable options for patients. There are a number of challenges to fixed salary compensation plans. Firstly, fixed salary models of compensation are also associated with a perverse incentive, namely that of undertreatment of patients. The inherent work ethic of faculty and their commitment to doing the right thing for patients is central to this model. Robust and engaged oversight by leadership is mandatory to ensure that patients are receiving proper care and that the work is equitably distributed. The lack of incentives may serve to keep a lid on clinical productivity which in effect can be suboptimal for patients who need the expertise of the unit and/or who need timely care. The challenges in driving productivity may lead to inefficient utilization of infrastructure and difficulty in driving needed revenue into the unit to cross-subsidize other missions and other resources that are important for faculty satisfaction (travel, etc.). The inability of surgeons to modulate their salary up or down is another substantial downside that may lead to dissatisfaction. While this is obvious on the upside, it can also be a problem for surgeons who would accept a reduction in pay in return for the ability to reduce their clinical activities.

Figure 14.2 depicts the most common compensation plan approach in Academic Medical Centers which combines elements of both (A) and (B) along with a defined incentive program. In this model receipts from the medical group (net of medical group and the Dean's taxes) and other salary supporting revenue (grants, medical directorships, etc.) flow through the department to cover department and divisional taxes, base salaries of the faculty, and other clinical and non-clinical expenses of the faculty member. In this model the residual profit or loss in essence belongs to the Department and not the faculty member. The department at its discretion may incorporate incentives on the basis of profitability of the individual faculty member, reaching certain levels of clinical activity (i.e. wRVU, cases, etc.), and/or other desired academic metrics. In this model there are many decisions which leaders must make including the level of departmental/divisional taxation, the methodology by which base salaries are set, the eligibility for participation in the incentive plan,

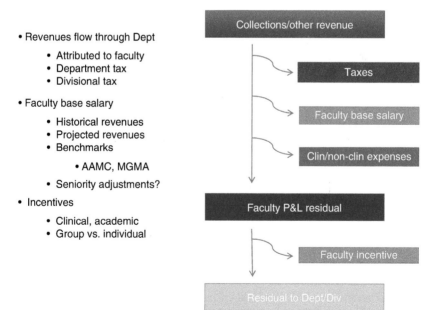

Fig. 14.2 Typical model of compensation in AMC

which incentives will be included, and what will occur with the residual profit or loss. Department taxation rates are generally based on budget expectations with respect to anticipated expenditures for central infrastructure perhaps with an extra margin included. Departments may choose to tax different revenue streams at different levels. For example, they may choose to tax clinical receipts at 10% while at the same time deciding not to levy taxes on purchased service revenues (medical directorships, grant support, etc.). In larger departments the divisions (subunits of the department) may also levy operational taxes to cover division-specific expenditures. The methodology by which the base salary is set is very institution-dependent. Many programs will set base salary at a certain benchmark percentile with some flexibility to go higher than this dependent upon local markets, necessary retentions, etc. There are a number of specialty-specific benchmark survey reports including the AAMC (Association of American Medical Colleges), the MGMA (Medical Group Management Association), SullivanCotter, Medscape, and others. Almost all of these survey reports are acquired by the institution through participation and the payment of institutional fees. The survey reports include tables by specialty and also by region. Under the licensing agreements, they are made available to management leaders of participating institutions for use in guiding salary decisions. While helpful in getting a feel for national and regional scales, there are a number of challenges to their use. One issue lies in the significant sub-specialization that exists within academic medical centers and the heterogeneity of non-clinical efforts that faculty are engaged in. This often precludes having adequate sample sizes in the survey for certain specialties/phenotypes. Not all surveys account for seniority in academic rank or for high level administrative responsibilities. The benchmark surveys also do not adequately factor in the heterogeneity (or performance level) of various efforts (research, clinical, administrative, etc.) Notwithstanding, the benchmark surveys can be useful in identifying conservative minimum base salary levels that can then be augmented by individual faculty specific considerations such as prior year receipts, the presence of substantive non-clinical salary support revenues, and premiums for recruitment and retention. It is important to apply consistency to this process.

A further nuance in the construction of compensation plans in traditional academic medical centers lies in the recent trend towards integration of the medical group and medical center to create different funds flow models. The impetus for this arose out of the increasing difficulty that departments faced in being profitable secondary to declining professional fees, increased practice expenses, and the challenging funding environment. In this model as depicted in Fig. 14.3 and as outlined in Chap. 13, the clinical salary supporting revenues are in the form of care payments instead of professional billing receipts. Clinical practice expenses are borne by the health system and the professional billing receipts flow to the integrated health system. The health system then flows to the departments (purchased service agreement) a payment for the care rendered. The care payment in most academic medical centers are currently work-RVU based and rely upon specialty specific benchmark surveys such as the MGMA dollar per work RVU tables. From this revenue the department/division pays faculty salaries (including base and incentives) and other

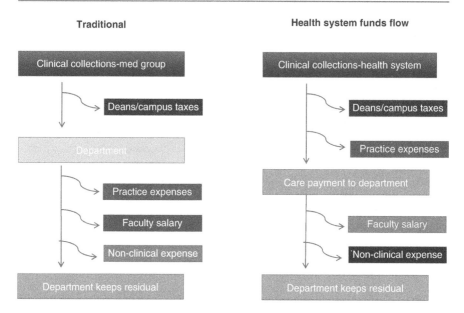

Fig. 14.3 Funds flow model: integrated health system

clinical and non-clinical expenses. There are a few challenges to such plans. For example, providers from different specialties will generate different levels of revenue (because the specialty specific $/wRVU rates differ) for performing the same procedure. For example ENT surgeons and general surgeons will drive different care payment levels for performing a thyroidectomy. Neurosurgeons and general vascular surgeons will generate different revenues for a carotid endarterectomy. Some departments will pool the care payments and attribute the same carepayment rate to all of their surgeons for each wRVU generated. An important nuance in the funds flow models that affect the amount of revenue available for faculty salary revolves around what expenses are left inside the departments and divisions. For example, in many institutions that employ a funds flow model, mid-level providers are left on the books of the department. Most mid-level providers in surgical units are facilitators of faculty clinical activity without substantial independent billing and thus may greatly reduce the pool of dollars available to the faculty compensation plan.

Transparency and Monitoring

Another sensitive issue that arises in the development of compensation plans revolves around transparency. Some faculty have the perception that compensation decisions occur in a smoky backroom with a degree of capriciousness and perhaps favoritism. Many public institutions display the compensation of their employees including their surgeons in online databases that are accessible to the general public (including your peers). Even in those institutions that do not, it would be unwise to think that faculty do not communicate with each other regarding their packages. While it is critical that surgical leadership be able to rationally defend all compensation decisions as the product of consistent methodology, there will always be sensitivities such that complete transparency and public commentary of individual faculty salary levels is generally unwise (in my opinion). Notwithstanding, it is critical that the process be generally transparent. Faculty will in general recognize that variations in activity portfolios and performance levels will lead to some heterogeneity in pay. Minimizing variations that are not related to overall activity levels and performance is critical though. This includes to some extent the issue of seniority. Modest salary differentials associated with seniority are well tolerated whereas substantial pay differences despite similar portfolios of activities are not.

Monitoring of the compensation plan in regular intervals is critical to the financial viability of these programs and in ensuring that the plan is functioning well with respect to achieving the desired characteristics as established by the governance. This is best done by a compensation committee or an executive group that includes the business officer, the department's vice-chairs for finance and faculty affairs, the Chair, and a few others. The monitoring strategy should focus on reviewing the overall financial situation, on outliers on the high and low-end of incentives, and on major themes of parity such as gender equity.

Conclusions

The development and implementation of surgery faculty compensation plans is amongst the most important of responsibilities that department and divisional leaders will engage in. Through these plans you will drive your priorities and in very real ways, you will impact the lives of those that you are tasked with stewarding. The conversations with faculty surrounding compensation will on many occasions be very difficult. While it might seem convenient to direct faculty salary inquiries and concerns to the department business manager, the most effective surgical leaders insinuate themselves instead and see these meetings as opportunities to listen, learn, educate, and motivate. Leaders that are perceived by faculty to be insensitive to their concerns and needs in this area are set up to fail and will have difficulty driving performance and change.

Negotiating: How, When and Why

15

T. Clark Gamblin and Timothy M. Pawlik

The subject of negotiating in the work place often conjures images of power struggles and leveraging to obtain more resources and/or support. In reality, negotiating is not an event, but rather a process. From the moment that each day begins, we must consider tradeoffs and negotiate where to invest our time. While contracts are important, contracts are only a small part of negotiating in the workplace. As individuals seek resources, higher pay, and greater job opportunities, it is important to realize that negotiating with supervisors begins when you are first hired, occurs each day, and continues until the employment ends.

When negotiating, four outcomes are generally possible. The first is a "win–win" where both parties feel that they have been heard and values the decision as mutually beneficial. This type of outcome should always occur as part of a faculty recruitment. If a faculty feels the letter of offer grossly undervalues him/her or leadership feels that they have pushed beyond the value of the recruit, the partnership will suffer and likely fail. The second outcome is a "win–lose" result. In this situation, one party feels that they have secured an advantageous resolution while the other party feels they have not gained. This situation is sustainable only if the "lose" party recognizes an unanticipated return or the next interaction compensates for the selflessness in the preceding deal. The third outcome is a "lose–lose" result in which both parties refuse to yield and the lack of agreement is detrimental to both. Finally, a fourth negotiating

T. C. Gamblin
Division of Surgical Oncology, Department of Surgery, Medical College of Wisconsin, Milwaukee, WI, USA
e-mail: tcgamblin@mcw.edu

T. M. Pawlik (✉)
Department of Surgery, The Ohio State University, Wexner Medical Center, Columbus, OH, USA
e-mail: Tim.Pawlik@osumc.edu

outcome can be no progress or an agreement is reached with both parties moving along with neither being negatively impacted. This neutral/no progress result offers limited downside and if no hard feelings exist, can be revisited.

Ingredients for success in negotiation includes time, information and power. Each should be carefully considered and measured to optimize the results. Negotiating time is often without a clear beginning or end and is a continuous process. It has been said that the value of the agreement is often equal to the time and effort invested. Formal details in any negotiating process often conclude in the last 20% of the allotted time, and thus patience typically pays off. Information is incredibly valuable and approaching a negotiating meeting to just discover what the other party has to say or propose is potentially a lost opportunity. It is a risk knowing less information than your counterpart and therefore prepared individuals anticipate the data needed and arrive well prepared. Discovery type approaches when meeting with a counterpart are challenging because interests, needs and motivation are often concealed in face-to-face meetings, making discovery of valuable information unlikely. One potential approach is to speak to others who have negotiated with your counterpart before, particularly if you are approaching this person on a similar issue such as salary, support, or research space.

Power is the ability to influence situations and/or people. Although some consider "power" a negative term, it is not. Power does not imply that one side necessarily dominates the other side. Some power comes from a formal position, for example a department chair or a dean. Other power is linked to expertise and insight into a situation. The ability to provide incentives or punishments has also been associated with power. In addition, passion and charisma can provide confidence and power in some deliberations. Lack of interest/apathy is often an overlooked form of power. For example, a car buyer who does not want to buy a car today holds substantial power; also, the home buyer who does not want to debate over the sale price holds power. In some cases, bizarre and irrational behavior can also confer tremendous amounts of power, but if unprofessional or mistimed can also lead to premature ending of the negotiation process. Powerful people generally have high self-esteem. One important technique to gain self-esteem and become powerful is through preparation. Power in a negotiation is, however, often more balanced than it appears and seldom is completely one sided. Power in relationships can change as individuals establish where they are willing to go and when they will push back. Power should be tested carefully to understand what is available.

Questioning skills are essential in negotiating. It is best to have insightful, relevant, and focused questions prepared. Goals of your questions should include knowing the other party's motivations and interest. Questions can be restrictive or expansive. Restrictive, closed ended questions seek granular information, direct the conversation and get dialogue started. Restrictive questions can also confirm a critical point or be used to gain concession. Expansive, open ended questions, gain more information, reveal behavioral styles, and allow for listening. By asking lots of questions the other party feels valued and heard. Questions can also help fill in gaps of knowledge by providing clarity and verifying information, as well as be used to check the understanding of your counterpart and their level of interest. By using phrases like "Were you aware …", information can be shared in a nonthreatening manner while using an engaging question. Some questions can also be used to redirect someone's attention using such phrases as "Can we get back to …". Agreement may sometimes be reached more quickly by using such phrases as "Would you be willing to consider …" Questions help your counterpart feel they have participated in the solution. In addition, phrases such as "You seem opposed to …, why?" may be enlightening and a catalyst for more conversation.

In order to gain accurate information, have a goal and plan for the interaction. Try to understand what motivates your counterpart and realize if they are a task oriented individual or more of a people person/relationship oriented individual. Understanding this difference helps focus on how quickly to approach the issues at hand and how personal individuals will take tense or direct conversations. Questioning should move from broad to narrow issues and involve an organized manner to understand the agenda and the culture. Improper timing of questions may limit information or even end the conversation. Responses are best linked to the next questions and silence is valuable and important. Stop talking and listen to your counterpart. In addition, taking notes at the time of the discussion can help with recall and is often felt to demonstrate interest in your counterpoint's comments.

It is common to not listen well in negotiating and this often leads to important missed opportunities. Poor listeners are often inaccurate and/or incomplete in their recall. The goal is to maintain objectivity and try to understand the goals of the other individual. This understanding can only be accomplished with effective observation and listening. Most effective listeners will uncover additional needs and goals. Other pitfalls of negotiating include the misconception that negotiating is primarily persuasion. It is not, and therefore it doesn't require talking all the time; rather, negotiating is as much as about understanding the motivations of another person in order to influence. Concentrating on what to say next rather than listening to what is being said is a common mistake and can limit understanding and your ability to be a good negotiator. Emotions can also limit observations and impressions seen with nonverbal and vocal intonation.

Attentive listening is hard work and requires motivation, thoughtful questions and alertness to nonverbal cues. Allow your counterpart to tell their story first as this shows respect and also allows for the ability to adjust and modify your own thoughts based on information gained. As a counterpart shares their story or point, do not interrupt them even if the information is not correct, as they should be allowed to finish speaking. Interruptions should be minimized. Phones should be silenced and doors closed to decreased distractions. Always look your counterpart in the eyes and give undivided attention. When interacting, react only to the message and not the person and never slip into a personal debate. Anger often interferes with problem solving and internal control must be maintained.

Preparation for negotiation is critical for success and maximizes the potential that both parties will be satisfied with the results. Corners should not be cut in preparation and initial meetings held to "listen and discover issues" without data are not helpful and likely may yield to a suboptimal outcome. Prior to the meeting, the purpose of the meeting must be clearly defined and an ideal outcome should be identified. Preparation not only includes data but also seeking insight of others. A strong preparation includes considering the explicit and implicit needs of your counterpart. Negotiable flexible issues should be privately outlined and readied for discussion as needed. Questions prior to negotiation include; who will be present, what is the counterpart style and what alternatives exist. Most negotiating will lead to future negotiations with the same person and this must be an important consideration.

Every individual should establish a private Best Alternative to a Negotiated Agreement (BATNA) prior to initiating a negotiation. This BATNA scenario is the next best solution to what one hopes from deliberation. During this phase, one should question what happens if "walking away" occurs. Focusing on what can be done to gain a counterpart's cooperation and if discussions break down a meditator may help. In some cases, location may influence an outcome and meeting a counterpart in their office setting may help the counterpart feel respected, valued and comfortable. Outlining an agenda prior to the meeting also offers clarity for what is planned and may allow parties to prepare while reducing the unknown. Discussions should be interactive to ensure understanding and provide clarity. Questions such as "Precisely, what do you mean?" allow an interactive agenda. Verification can be obtained as well with statements such as "As I understand …". Empathy in the discussion may allow parties to connect and reflective listening acknowledges emotions and shares content back and forth in an attempt to gain consensus. It may be best to be noncommittal early in discussions with statements such as " It sounds like …" and "It appears that ….".

Most negotiations are based on body language and tone even more than the actual words. Not only is body language important to match with the message but also to interpret the counterpart's nonverbal actions and discern their position. Many nonverbal approaches can occur and acute awareness of your counterpart is valuable. Body language such as leaning forward symbolizes some element of agreement, while shifting weight and leaning backwards may signal disagreement. Arms folded or over the back of the chair often show lack of receptiveness. Open palms generally signify transparency while touching one's face and wringing hands may represent nervousness. Crossed legs may signify a lack of cooperation and trust. Generally, feet flat on the floor is the most effective stance. Nonverbals should be considered in clusters rather than as a single signal.

Building trust is essential to obtain even minor concessions and concessions will be incredibly difficult if trust is not strong. Keys to build such trust include the ability to demonstrate expertise and articulate interest and support of the negotiation process. Nonverbals must match what is being said verbally to maximize outcomes. Intentions to satisfy both parties should be clearly communicated and reliability represents a long-term potential. Listening to obtain complete information should occur prior to giving any opinions. Discussions should address difficult items directly and provide accurate data. Patience with deliberate slow speaking is important and being open to calculated risks shows cooperation. If the counterpart is not trustworthy, negotiations often must still occur. Terms should be spelled out in details and time lines should be defined. Details may also include rewards/penalties for success and/or nonperformance. In certain cases, a third party may be helpful to mediate. Trust is reciprocal and if one party signals distrust it leads to potential destruction on both sides.

Great negotiators create mutual beneficial deals and plan for the infinite, never operating in a vacuum. Successful negotiators create positivity, know their subject well, and have a firm grasp on the process. Using the same style of negotiations in all situations is a habit that could be viewed as lazy, unintelligent and even arrogant. Because counterparts are different, such an approach will not yield consistent results. Counterparts should be approached in their comfort zone which is dependent on their personality, the stakes and the culture. Styles are important to understand both through introspective inspection, as well as study of your counterpart. Cordial negotiators are good listeners, trusting, want harmony, and have a strong need to feel recognized and valued. Personable approaches tend to yield the most productive results. "Results" negotiators tend to be impatient, view others as adversaries and value the outcome more than feelings. "Analytic" negotiators need timely accurate data, minimize personal feelings, process slowly, and cautiously ask lots of questions. "Blended" negotiators tend to be flexible, keep things light, are personable/social and tend to build team with creative approaches. Steps to identify the optimal style should include awareness of surroundings such the counterpart's office setup and asking probing questions.

In summary, negotiations occur constantly and planning is essential to maximize the outcome for both parties. Preparation with adjusted style and body language are essential for success. Using intuition alone is not as effective as a planned approach and negotiation is learned skill. Listening, building trust and compromise are the keys to success in most negotiations.

How Cultures Influence Leadership Styles

16

Marco G. Patti and Daniel Albo

Introduction

In 1994, for the first time in the history of the American College of Surgeons (ACS), an individual who was not born in the United States (US) and had not trained in the US, was elected President. In his Presidential address delivered during the 78th Convocation of the ACS on October 13, 1994 Dr. Alexander J. Walt stated: "*I stand here as the first foreign medical graduate (FMG) to be President of this College…….* *The election of a FMG testifies to the great generosity of our American Society, to its warmth, tolerance, acceptance of strangers, willingness to experiment, and its disdain for artificial barriers……*" [1]. Nineteen years later, on October 6, 2013 another FMG, Carlos A. Pellegrini, gave his Presidential address in front of 1622 new fellows of the College as the 94th President. Of the 1622 initiates, 346 (21.3%) were from 55 countries around the world. Even though Dr. Walt and Dr. Pellegrini are examples that are difficult to follow, their stories have a lot in common and show that foreign-born individuals do serve in leadership roles in surgery.

Foreign Medical Graduates (FMG)

In 2017, a study based on the National Residency Matching Program statistics, published the trends in the proportion of students who matched into categorical general surgery (GS) residency positions. During the period between 1994 and 2014, they showed a steadily decrease (at a rate of one-half percentage point each year) of GS

M. G. Patti (✉)
Medicine and Surgery, University of North Carolina, Chapel Hill, NC, USA
e-mail: marco_patti@med.unc.edu

D. Albo
Department of Surgery, Medical College of Georgia, Augusta, GA, USA
e-mail: DALBO@augusta.edu

© Springer Nature Switzerland AG 2019
M. R. Kibbe, H. Chen (eds.), *Leadership in Surgery*, Success in Academic Surgery, https://doi.org/10.1007/978-3-030-19854-1_16

postgraduate-first year (PGY1) positions occupied by US seniors. However, during the same period, they proved that these GS positions have been filled by US FMG and non-US FMG applicants [2].

While some of them were American citizens, the majority were born and educated abroad. It is very important to separate these two groups. Generally, American citizens attended school and college in the US and then enrolled in a medical school abroad, mostly because they could not secure a position in one of the 151 accredited medical degree programs in the US. After graduation, and after passing the required exams (i.e., the United States Medical Licensing Examination [USMLE]), they eventually obtained a residency position in the US. In contrast, the majority of FMGs were born and raised abroad, and went to school, college, medical school and sometimes even completed a residency in their own countries. For them the path to a residency position in the US is very cumbersome, as it involves learning a new language, passing the USMLE exams, and often doing a couple of years of research in the US before applying for a residency position. In fact, there is no reciprocal recognition of training between the US and the rest of the world, so that even surgeons who are board certified in their own countries must complete a residency in the US in order to be eligible for board certification and independent practice [3, 4]. It is a long and hard process that requires many sacrifices: 1) leaving their own country, their family, and their friends; 2) facing expenses for the multiple examinations (around $3000) that are often equivalent to a 1 year salary in many underdeveloped countries [5]; and finally, 3) being immersed in an social and professional environment that is often radically different from their own. Language, beliefs, and family structure are unique to the American culture. For instance, in many other countries the role of the doctor is completely different, more "god-like". Similarly, the role of nurses and other health care professionals, the concepts of informed consent, confidentiality, and documentation are unique to the American health care system [6].

So why are so many individuals willing to undergo this long process and make considerable sacrifices? There are indeed some very strong personal and professional reasons. The US is still seen as a land of opportunity. It is seen as a unique place in the world where an immigrant can become educated and wealthy, and where meritocracy is still the norm rather than the exception. Thus, there is a strong desire for many to try to achieve a comfortable economic situation, guaranteeing an education and a better future for their own children. In addition, there are some characteristics of the surgical education in the US that are absolutely distinctive: it is a system that is open minded, flexible, grants graded responsibility, and practices a hands-on approach. In contrast to many other countries where training periods extend to 10–15 years before a surgeon is considered ready for independent practice, in the US a general surgeon is produced in 5 years, a neurosurgeon in 7 years, and a cardio-thoracic surgeon in 7–8 years. And contrary to many other countries, employment is a certainty after completion of training.

Due to the shortage of American-born applicants to General Surgery programs, the number of FMGs will increase overtime. It is therefore important to understand and respect the cultural differences that exist. For the world of surgery it is a unique opportunity to create a work force characterized by the blending of many different cultures that will better serve a country blossoming with diversity.

In this chapter, we will focus on the influence of culture on leadership. We will use the term FMG to indicate individuals who were born and educated abroad before doing their residency in the US.

Leadership

There are many definitions of leadership. Wikipedia defines leadership "... *as a process of social influence in which one person can enlist the aid and support of others in the accomplishment of a common task....*" [7]. Patel et al. identified qualities that are essential for leaders in the area of surgery [8]:

- **Professionalism**. Leaders must be honest, ethical and serve as a role model for their team.
- **Technically competence**. Leaders must be recognized by their team as competent surgeons.
- **Motivation**. Leaders must have clear goals and expectations in order to motivate their team.
- **Innovation**. Leaders should have a vision and be able to adopt new ideas.
- **Teamwork**. Leaders should be able to create and lead a team with a common goal.
- **Communication skills**. Leaders should be able to convey information to others so that they understand the goal.
- **Decision making**. Leaders should be able to choose the best options and take responsibility, even when the situation is not certain.
- **Emotional competence**. Leaders should be able to control his/her own emotions and those of others.
- **Resilience**. A leader should be able to adjust and recover from setbacks and changes to achieve a designated goal.
- **Effective teaching**. A leader should be able to transfer knowledge and skills to others.

Some feel that individuals are born with inherited traits which determine leadership [9], while others think that individuals can learn to become leaders through teaching and observation [10]. We believe that what makes a leader is probably a combination of the two. Leadership, in fact, is influenced by many factors:

- **Generations**: Today, the majority of the individuals in leadership positions belong to the baby boom generation. Baby boomers are goal-oriented, hardworking, and driven to success. They value power, and believe in a hierarchical system. Members of generation X are very heterogeneous in terms of race, religion and ethnicity. They respect talent more than authority, and for them worklife balance is a priority. In contrast, generation Y (the leaders of the future) have a sense of entitlement, do not believe in hierarchy, and demand to be mentored and to achieve an ideal balance between work and private life.

- **Gender**. Although medicine has historically been a male-dominated profession, the Association of American Medical Colleges (AAMC) reported that during the last years, female presence has been steadily increasing, with women representing half (50.1%) of medical school matriculates in 2017 [11]. Conversely, while the number of women entering medicine has been increasing, there is still a significant underrepresentation of women in faculty and leadership positions in medicine. In 2015, women made up 39% of faculty, but only 22% held full professorship, with 23% tenured [12].
- **Race**. Health care disparities according to race and ethnicity remain a persistent and insidious problem. Despite efforts to promote diversity in surgery, Blacks and Hispanics continue to be underrepresented [13]. In 2017, Abelson JS et al. performed a cross-sectional and longitudinal analysis providing an updated description of diversity along the academic surgical pipeline. It was shown that in 2014–2015, 12.4% of the American citizens were represented by the black population. However, they represented only 5.7% of graduating medical students, 6.2% of general surgery trainees, 3.8% of assistant professors, 2.5% of associate professors and 2.0% of full professors. In addition, from 2005 to 2015, representation among Black associate professors has worsened (0.07%/year, $p < 0.01$) [14]. Thus, while the U.S. population is growing increasingly diverse, this study demonstrates that this increase is not reflected in our medical school graduates, surgical trainees, and academic surgical workforce.
- **Mentorship**. Mentors can help facilitate professional and personal development with respect to leadership skills thorough an assessment of strengths and weakness, helping in tasks such as decision-making, diplomacy, and conflict resolution.
- **Upbringing**. It is easier to become a leader when the focus of the educational process has been to eventually assume a position of leadership. This is based on solid role models, often within the same family, and constant positive reinforcement.
- **Culture**. There is no question that culture influences leadership. While this is not an issue for individuals who are born and raised in the country where they work, it plays an important role for individuals who were born and raised in a country different from the one where they eventually decide to live and work.

Culture and Leadership

Culture stems from ethnicity, language, beliefs, religion, customs, and philosophy of life. Different groups of human beings who live in different areas of the world are distinguished from one another by cultural traits, and this determines cultural diversity. Two concepts are closely related to culture and leadership: ethnocentrism and prejudice.

- **Ethnocentrism** is the tendency to favor one's own culture (race or ethnicity) over others, valuing one's own beliefs and attitudes over those of others. This is a major obstacle to effective leadership as it can prevent a leader from understanding and valuing other people's cultures. It can also make individuals less tolerant of other people's behaviors. For instance, a leader that grew up in a culture that respects hierarchy and authority may find it difficult to deal with somebody that challenges his/her authority
- **Prejudice** is a negative attitude toward individuals or members of a group, based on one's own beliefs and feelings rather than on objective facts. Prejudice results from having an ethnocentric behavior. Classic examples are prejudices about race, gender, sexual orientations, and religion.

Many studies have focused on national culture and on what distinguishes one society or a nation from another, the so called "dimensions of culture" [15, 16]. Geert Hofstede identified five dimensions that distinguish societies [15]:

1. **Power distance index**. The extent to which members of an organization accept that power is not distributed equally.
2. **Individualism vs. collectivism**. The degree by which people prefers to act as individuals rather than group members.
3. **Masculinity vs. femininity**. The degree by which ideals such as competition and success (masculine ideals) are valued over caring for others and quality of life, traditionally considered "feminine" ideals.
4. **Uncertainty avoidance**. The degree by which a group uses norms and procedures to make the future more certain.
5. **Long-term orientation**. The degree by which goals are set for long-term objectives rather than for immediate gratification.

Another very important cross-cultural comparison study was the so called Global Leadership and Organizational Behavior Effectiveness (GLOBE) project [16]. The data in this study came from questionnaire responses from 17,000 managers in 62 countries. Globe identified nine cultural dimensions, adding four to the work of Hofstede.

6. **Gender egalitarianism**. The degree by which a group minimizes gender inequality.
7. **Assertiveness**. The level of confrontation and aggressiveness versus harmony and solidarity.
8. **Performance orientation**. The degree by which individuals in a group are rewarded for improvement and excellence.
9. **In-group collectivism**. The degree by which individuals express pride and loyalty to the organization and family.

Based on similarities in these dimensions, GLOBE divided nations into ten main cultural clusters, based on the belief that cultures are formed around regions that

Table 16.1 Cultural clusters

Cluster	Countries
Nordic Europe	Denmark, Norway, Finland
Germanic Europe	Germany, Austria, the Netherlands
Latin Europe	Italy, Spain, Portugal, France, Israel, Switzerland
Eastern Europe	Slovenia, Poland, Hungary, Russia, Georgia, Greece, Albania
Anglo	US, United Kingdom, Ireland, Canada, Australia, South Africa-white, New Zealand
Latin America	Argentina, Bolivia, Chile, Colombia, Ecuador, Paraguay, Peru, Uruguay, Venezuela
Southern Asia	Indonesia, Malaysia, Thailand, India, Philippines
Confucian Asia	China, South Korea, Japan, Singapore
Middle East	Turkey, Egypt, Morocco, Kuwait
Sub-Saharan Africa	Nigeria, South Africa-black, Zambia, Zimbabwe

share common historical, political, economic and environmental backgrounds (Table 16.1). The study clearly identified differences among these ten cultural clusters. For instance, while in the Nordic Europe cluster gender egalitarianism and institutional collectivism were very strong, in the Middle East cluster gender egalitarianism was very low as women are usually afforded less status than men and are rarely in a position of leadership.

The goal of the GLOBE project was to see how different cultures determined different approaches to leadership. Six different leadership styles were identified:

- **Charismatic**. Leadership reflects the ability to inspire and motivate.
- **Team oriented**. Leadership emphasizes team building and common goals.
- **Participative**. Leadership emphasizes involvement of others in decision making and a non-autocratic behavior.
- **Human-oriented**. Leadership that is characterized by compassion, generosity, and sensitivity to other people's needs.
- **Autonomous**. Leadership that is individualistic and autocratic.
- **Self-protective**. Self-centered leadership, status conscious and face saving.

Relating to the clusters described before, it is easy to identify a leadership style for each cluster. For instance, a Confucian Asia leadership style is team oriented but at the same time the leader uses status and position to make decisions independently, without the input of others. In contrast, in Anglo countries the leaders want to be non-autocratic, team-oriented and considerate of others. And they believe that face saving represents ineffective leadership.

Overall the study identified positive leadership attributes (confidence building, honesty, excellence-oriented, and motivational) and negative attributes (autocratic, non-cooperative, asocial, irritable). Clearly people from most cultures think that good leadership is based on integrity, charisma, and interpersonal skills.

In summary, this study underlines the intricacies of leadership and how it is influenced by culture. Furthermore, the GLOBE project stresses the importance of abandoning our ethnocentric behavior and opening our mind to different perspectives, with the goal of developing a richer understanding of the leadership process.

The FMG and the American Training System

As mentioned before, the path is very long for a FMG to get into an American residency program, often the end-result of a process that can take anywhere between 3 and 7 years. Most FMGs enjoy tremendously the training period. Even if they have completed a residency in surgery before, they treasure the teaching in pre- and post-operative care, the multi-disciplinary approach to the care of the patient, the progressive independency in the operating room, the evolving role as teachers for those who come after them. There is no question that at the beginning of the training, the FMGs feel a sense of pressure, the need to prove to themselves and the people that put their trust in them that it was not a mistake. The completion of training brings a unique sense of relief, the realization that it was possible to function at the same level as an American medical graduate and succeed in a different system.

As the end of the residency gets closer, however, the FMG has to make an important decision, something that has a tremendous impact in his/her future, both personally and professionally. It is the difficult choice between securing a job in the US and starting a path toward citizenship versus going back to the country of origin. Clearly it is a balance between different powerful forces. On one side, there is the realization that working in the US is very gratifying. As shown by the example of others who have reached the pinnacle of American surgery, the US system allows the individual to reach his/her full potential and to be rewarded for hard and high quality work. Along with the professional satisfaction, there is the certainty of an economically safe life, with the possibility of providing opportunities and an education to their own children, something often not possible in their country of origin. On the other hand, there is the realization that staying in the US means to be away from family, friends, habits, and life style as it was. In a way, it depends on the degree of assimilation that has occurred during the years of training. Some FMGs have chosen **integration**, the conscious decision to accept different rules as a need to function in a culture different from their own, a culture that is not embraced, with preservation of their own values. This is typified by the FMG that goes home after work and spend time only with members of his/her own cultural group, speaking the language of their childhood, trying to raise his/her own children if they were not in the US. In such a situation the individual feels a tremendous pressure and lives a dichotomous life, American while at work, foreigner when at home. For other FMGs a slow process of **assimilation** occurs during training. It is based on the acceptance of new values, different beliefs, and a different life style. For a person who has only reached a state of integration, there is often the regret of "what life could have been" if he/she went back to their country of origin after completion of training in the US. However, the person who has been slowly and consciously assimilated into the US culture lives without regrets, enjoying the newly acquired status.

Clearly these different emotional situations have a very profound effect on the way the person will behave if in a position of leadership. The person who tries to hold on his/her own culture will try to impose the values and characteristics of two different worlds, often failing and creating tension in the work place environment.

In contrast, the individual fully or partially assimilated in the American system will show a leadership style that conforms to the "Anglo cluster" previously described. This person enjoys his/her acquired position and is grateful to the system, frequently trying to help others along the same difficult path.

Some of these concepts are better explained by personal examples.

From Italy to the US

I was born and raised in Catania, a town on the east coast of Sicily. After completing high school (there is no college in Italy), at age 18 I enrolled in medical school, one of 1500 new students who aspired to become physicians. I completed medical school at the top of my class, and I was accepted in the General Surgery program at the Vittorio Emanuele II hospital in Catania. Needless to say, I was enthusiastic about this choice. I was motivated by the desire to become a competent surgeon and by the ability of making a difference in other people's lives. The enthusiasm and the dreams, however, were short lived as I soon realized that the system was not designed to prepare one for an independent practice before age 45–50. The Chairman of the Department of Surgery performed all the difficult cases, leaving very little to other faculty members and residents. Interestingly, he had trained in the United States where he had enjoyed very much the educational system. Back in Sicily, however, he felt he could not change the culture of the place and went back to the dictatorial and autocratic system that he had left (please note that I always refer to male figures as there were no female faculty or female residents). There was no formal mentoring or teaching, and we mostly learned by observing, reading, and performing simple cases. Needless to say, I soon became disillusioned and I looked for a way to escape this reality. This presented in the form of a fellowship that supported research abroad. With the blessing of my Chairman, I applied and was accepted for a 1-year research position at the University of California San Francisco (UCSF). There I worked under the guidance of Lawrence W. Way and Carlos A. Pellegrini. I have to confess that the cultural shock was tremendous, and I am not only talking about the different language. Professionally, I soon realized I was in another world. Even though both Drs. Way and Pellegrini were very busy surgeons, they were always available for meetings during which they took the time to teach the intricacies of research, from formulating a hypothesis to designing an experiment to test it. But what struck me even more was the way resident education was structured. Interns and junior residents were taken through simple cases, while senior and chief residents were performing complex procedures. Residents were given progressive responsibility for patient care and Chief residents managed their services and were treated as junior colleagues by the faculty. This world was present and close, but yet incredibly far away for a foreigner. One year of research became 3 years, and after passing the required examinations, I applied through the National Residency Matching Program. In June of 1986, I started all over again as an intern in General Surgery at UCSF.

I have wonderful memories of the years I spent training: it was hard work but it was incredibly gratifying. Every day I felt I was learning something new, becoming a better physician. After graduation I was sent by Dr. Haile Debas (the Chairman at UCSF at that time) to train at the Queen Mary Hospital in Hong Kong with Professor John Wong. I went with one of the Chief Residents who graduated with me in 1993. Still, today, I remember my colleague's reaction to being immersed in a very hierarchical and autocratic system, and how he demanded things rather than earning them. While for him it was a real cultural shock, I adapted really fast and enjoyed my time!

After going back to UCSF, I spent the following 14 years working at Moffitt-Long Hospital as junior partner to Dr. L. W. Way (Carlos Pellegrini had moved to Seattle to become Chair of the Department of Surgery). Looking back, I can only be incredibly grateful to Dr. Way for his mentoring. He took a well-trained but rough individual and overtime he transformed him into a surgeon. I also treasured the continuous, albeit long distance, mentorship that Dr. Carlos Pellegrini has provided over the years, making sure that I excelled in other aspects of academic surgery, such as scholarship and leadership in surgical societies.

In 2008, I accepted the offer of Dr. Jeff Matthews, and moved to the University of Chicago where I assumed the position of Director of the Center for Esophageal Diseases. This was indeed a major honor, as I was trying to continue the tradition of Drs. David Skinner and Tom DeMeester, resuscitating a program that had been slowly dying after their departure [17].

In 2013 I married Dr. Melina R. Kibbe, a vascular surgeons who was working at Northwestern University in Chicago. In 2016, when she became the Chair of Surgery at the University of North Carolina, I moved to Chapel Hill, the third institution in my academic journey. And here I am enjoying working in a great public Institution, in a department led by a dynamic and dedicated chair who is driven by a sincere desire to have her faculty excel in the tripartite mission of academic medicine—clinical, education and research. In addition, I am enjoying a different quality of life, confirming that (as I always thought), it is not about "work-life balance" but rather "work-life choices".

Overall, if I look back and examine this 35-year journey, from Catania to Chapel Hill, what have I learned? How has this experience affected the way I lead other people?

- I have learned the value of hard work and resilience.
- I have learned to appreciate traits such as honesty and efficiency in delivering quality care to patients.
- I have set high standards for myself and for the people with whom I work.
- I have learned to recognize the importance of giving back, of mentoring others the way I was mentored. During the last 20 years, I have trained fellows from many continents. Some have gone back to their own country, while others have eventually followed my same path and remained in the US.

If I reflect on my own experience, I do not think that a complete process of assimilation has taken place, but rather the blending of two different cultures has occurred. From my original place of origin, I preserve the respect for authority, the respect for the elders, the gratitude for the tremendous opportunities I was given, and sometimes a feeling of annoyance when my authority is challenged by individuals who feel that things have to be given to them rather than earning them. From my country of adoption, I have learned the importance of embracing other cultures and be tolerant of differences, avoiding being ethnocentric, and be open to other people opinions with the goal of achieving a shared objective.

From Uruguay to the US

Although from Uruguay, I was a product of a mixture of the French and British system of medical training. In this type of system there is no college so that after high school (typically when 14–15 years old), you have to make a choice into a diversified pathway that is designed to lead you into a specific discipline. At this young age, many of my peers struggled with their decisions. For some reason, I always knew I wanted to be a Surgeon, so I chose the biological disciplines. Although the disadvantage of this system is that it forces people to make difficult and life-altering choices early on in their lives, it has the advantage of initiating profession-specific training at a much earlier age than in the US. Thus, it prepares you for life in Medical School and afterwards very effectively.

I entered Medical School in the top 3% and graduated from it in the top 1%. During my training years, I became an Instructor of Anatomy, a highly coveted position where a large number of students compete for one of ten positions available every year. The experiences of teaching Anatomy in Medical School at such a young age was a powerful influence in my career, as I learned early on that the best available way to learn is to teach others. After the required 6 years of Medical School training, I competed for one of the roughly 100 positions available in the country as an Intern, managing to enter in the top 3%. Eventually, I worked my way to a surgical House Staff officer position, where for 3 years I learned the intricacies of Surgery.

At this point, at the age of 25, I had to make a very difficult decision: stay home and fight an uphill battle, or leave my home country and come to the US. Like in Italy, Uruguay has a very autocratic and hierarchical system where you truly do not gain independence from your elders until your early to mid-forties. Not only that, but after so many years of relying on a competitive system to advance through the ranks, once you hit the job market, jobs in most private hospitals become very difficult to obtain without connections inside the system. Facing this reality, I married my lovely bride, Luisa, and we decided to come to the US for our grand adventure. We really did not have a clue as to what was in front of us, but there was no turning back.

Why the US? Like so many other FMGs, I was attracted by a system that can be best described as a meritocracy, as opposed to the autocracy that I was used to.

Simply put, in the US, if you are willing to sacrifice and commit to your development, you will have a shot at earning your way. That prospect was a very powerful driver that allowed us to push through what can be described as the trials of entrance into the US surgical training system, passing the NBME exams (today's USMLE exams) and eventually the two FLEX exams (they do not exist anymore) in order to be licensed.

Since the ACGME does not recognize surgical training abroad, I also had to repeat my surgical training. The challenge was to find a spot as a surgical resident. I reasoned that despite scoring very highly in my entrance exams, I was facing an uphill battle. Therefore, I decided to apply for a Surgical Research Fellowship position. Dr. Joel Roslyn, who I had briefly met in Uruguay while he was lecturing there, and who was moving from UCLA to the Medical College of Pennsylvania as a freshly minted Surgery Chairman, offered me a position as a Research Fellow. Dr. Roslyn not only gave me the opportunity to get started in the US, but he also became the most influential mentor in my career development; I will be forever grateful for his kindness, mentorship, and support. Under his guidance, our research laboratory became extremely productive and I was able to obtain a PhD degree in Molecular Pathobiology. This time in the lab became the platform that allowed me to eventually become a categorical resident at MCP-Hahnemann and it effectively launched my career as an academic surgeon in the US.

I absolutely loved my time in training and embraced it wholeheartedly. I was fascinated by the concentrated exposure to difficult disciplines, the system of progressive responsibility, and the emphasis on perioperative management. Above all, I loved the camaraderie with my fellow residents and the strong spirit de corps that we developed. We were, in the truest of ways, a team, and I knew that this was where I belonged. Unfortunately, shortly after MCP-Hahnemann became part of the AHERF system, AHERF went bankrupt. Simultaneously, Dr. Roslyn became ill and died way too young, cutting short a spectacular career in Academic Surgery. The residency program descended into severe turmoil and we all faced a difficult decision: to stay or to leave. True to my Hispanic heritage, where loyalty is a very important trait, I felt an enormous debt of gratitude to Dr. Roslyn, and decided to stay and finish what I felt we had started together. This was a unique experience since we had the opportunity of working very closely with the new Program Director in re-shaping our residency training program. In the most unlikely of circumstances, we all learned the powerful value of teamwork and of working together as one.

After residency, I was accepted for a 2-year fellowship in Surgical Oncology at MD Anderson. It was at Anderson where I learned the value of multidisciplinary care. It was a dream come true to be able to learn from some of the very brightest minds in the world of Oncology. After Anderson, I took my first job as faculty at the Medical College of Georgia, where we helped start a Surgical Oncology program and also participated in the creation of an MD/PhD Program in Oncology.

After Georgia, I accepted a job at Baylor College of Medicine initially as the Associate Operative Care Line Director for Operating Room activities at the MEDVAMC. This was my first experience in helping develop a matrix organization in healthcare. As a result of this matrix development our hospital moved from worst in the country in NSQIP outcomes to first, a remarkable testament to the power of collaborative teamwork. I was eventually promoted as the Vice Chairman and Director for Surgical Network Development as well as the Chief of General Surgery and Surgical Oncology.

After nearly 15 years in Houston, I moved back to the Medical College of Georgia as the Director for the Operative Care Line. This was a dream opportunity that I could not resist, since it gave me the opportunity of expanding a matrix organization style of management across an entire Cancer Center, The experience was so successful that eventually I was promoted as the Chair of the Department of Surgery at MCG as well as the Surgeon In Chief of the Health System. This platform has allowed me to help develop a matrix organization that now oversees all of the Perioperative Services across our large health care system.

In reflecting in all of this, my Hispanic cultural background values connectivity and relationships greatly, and I think this cultural influence heavily gravitated me to this wonderful healthcare matrix structures, one that develops multidisciplinary integrated health systems that are predicated in collaborative leadership and work across multiple silos. Ironically, In the process, I became the first Hispanic Chair of Surgery in the State of Georgia. Needless to say, at MCG we have embraced a culture of inclusivity and diversity that has enriched not only our Department of Surgery and our Cancer Center but the entire organization as well.

Along the way, I was very fortunate to become the first Hispanic president of the Association for Academic Surgery. I joined the AAS at a critical juncture in the life of this marvelous academic surgical society. It was at the AAS that I learned some of the most valuable lessons in collaborative leadership, and where I first realized that the whole is a lot more powerful than the sum of the parts. Over the last two decades, I have been blessed to work with truly amazing and passionate individuals. Together, we have embraced diversity like very few other societies have, and became an all-inclusive society with representation from people from all races, genders, and all walks of academic life. It is this diversity that helped transform the AAS into the vibrant and energetic dynamo that is today. It was the influx of fresh ideas and points of view that allowed the development of so many program-building new initiative such as the fall courses, the international academic career development courses, and other global health initiatives, and many more.

We are all the result of our collective upbringing, life experiences and mentorship. Together, these form a powerful cultural shaper that comes to define the frames that we use to see ourselves, and each other. When I reflect on how my experiences have helped develop my leadership style and qualities, I think the most important lessons that I learned are the willingness of embracing diversity and the force multiplying value of developing richly textured teams. Ultimately, it is all about building Programs, and allowing these programs to become the matrix where academic surgeons are nurtured and developed. In the process, I have gone from mentee to mentor of many of our students, residents, and faculty; I consider this awesome responsibility my most important job.

How Culture Impacts Leadership Styles in Surgery

We completed our training a couple of decades ago and during this time we have adapted to the "Anglo" style of leadership, in part as a necessity but mostly as the recognition that it is the best possible way to motivate others to follow and achieve a common goal. But as we look at each other and reflect on our careers, some common leadership traits emerge among us, the FMGs:

- FMGs tend to set high standards and be very hard on themselves. In terms of leadership style, this translates into the desire to lead by example and serve as a role model, by being honest and ethical, hard-working, and showing excellence in patient care both in operating room and on the ward.
- FMGs leaders tend to be less tolerant of those who expect things to be given to them without working hard to earn them.
- FMGs leaders have a desire to help others who share the same vision and goals.
- FMGs are often more embracing of differences than American born leaders. Having been exposed to prejudice themselves, FMG leaders they try to avoid it in their own work environment. Thus, a leadership style that is characterized by compassion, generosity, and sensitivity to other people's needs is common.
- FMGs leaders tend to have clear goals and expectations
- FMGs tend to lead by team building. They foster an environment designed to create consensus, rather than autocracy.
- Finally, based on their own life experience, FMGs are able to make decisions and take ultimate responsibility for them. They exhibit a leadership style characterized by decision making and resilience.

Conclusions

Culture affects leadership. The ideal end-result is achieved by those individuals who have been able to identify and blend the best characteristics of the two cultures, the one of their country of origin and that of the country where now they work and live. The responsibility of those who have gone down this path is to assist the FMGs who will come after them, making sure that they understand that while it is essential to focus on the destination, it is also important to enjoy the wonderful journey in the world of American surgery.

Acknowledgement   *Disclosure*: The Authors have no conflict of interest.

References

1. Walt AJ. The Uniqueness of American surgical education. Bull Am Coll Surg. 1994;79:9–20.
2. Are C, Stoddard H, Carpenter LA, O'Holleran B, Thompson JS. Trends in the match rate and composition of candidates matching into categorical general surgery residency positions in the United States. Am J Surg. 2017;213(1):187–94.

3. Cerio DR, Loghmanee CF. International medical graduates in American surgery: past, present, future. Bull Am Coll Surg. 2007;92:39–42.
4. McMahon GT. Coming to America – international medical graduates in the United States. N Engl J Med. 2004;350:24352437.
5. Lamb MN, Fraley DR. The Mayo Clinic-Rochester experience with IMGs as general surgery trainees. Surgery. 2006;140:351–3.
6. Whelan GP. Coming to America: the integration of International Medical Graduates into the American Medical Culture. Acad Med. 2005;81:176–8.
7. Leadership. https://en.wikipedia.org/wiki/Leadership.
8. Patel VM, Warren O, Humphris P, Ahmed K, Ashrafian H, rao C, Athanasiou T, Darzi A. What does leadership in surgery entail? ANZ J Surg. 2010;80:876–83.
9. Allport F, Allport GW. Personality traits: their classification and measurement. J Abnorm Soc Psychol. 1921;16:1–40.
10. Blake R, Mouton J. The managerial grid: the key to leadership excellence. Houston, TX: Gulf Publishing; 1964.
11. U.S. Medical School Applications and Matriculants by School, State of Legal Residence, and Sex, 2017-2018 [database on the Internet]. Available from: https://www.aamc.org/download/321442/data/factstablea1.pdf.
12. Benchmarking- full-time faculty by gender, rank, tenure [database on the Internet]. Available from: https://www.aamc.org/download/481194/data/2015table7.pdf; 2015.
13. Abelson JS, Wong NZ, Symer M, Eckenrode G, Watkins A, Yeo HL. Racial and ethnic disparities in promotion and retention of academic surgeons. Am J Surg. 2018;216:678. https://doi.org/10.1016/j.amjsurg.2018.07.020.
14. Abelson JS, Symer MM, Yeo HL, Butler PD, Dolan PT, Moo TA, Watkins AC. Surgical time out: our counts are still short on racial diversity in academic surgery. Am J Surg. 2018;215(4):542–8.
15. Hofstede G. Culture's consequences: comparing values, behaviors, institutions, and organizations across nations. Thousand Oaks, CA: Sage; 2001.
16. House RJ, Hanges PJ, Javidan M, Dorfman PW, Gupta V & Associates. Culture, leadership and organizations: the GLOBE study of 62 societies. Thousand Oaks: CA; Sage; 2004.
17. Greene LC, Worrell SG, Patti MG, DeMeester TR. The University of Chicago contribution to the treatment of gastroesophageal reflux disease and its complications. A tribute to David B. Skinner 1935-2003. Ann Surg. 2015;261:445. https://doi.org/10.1097/SLA.0698.

Women as Leaders in Surgery

17

Omaida C. Velazquez, Julie Ann Freischlag, and Diana Farmer

How Sex and Gender Impacts Leadership: Diana Farmer

Effective leaders are best described by their values and accomplishments. However, data shows an unfortunate alternative metric. A leader's sex or gender should reasonably have no expectation or consequence but there exists an unequivocal disparity in the number of male leaders compared to females. This can be attributed to the historical repercussions of centuries of beliefs that it was not a woman's role to serve as a leader, especially in the surgical field. Empirical research shows that the only difference in leadership style between sexes is that women tend to use a more democratic and transformational leadership style than their male counterparts [1] a value that is arguably more important than ever.

O. C. Velazquez (✉)
DeWitt Daughtry Family Department of Surgery, Leonard M. Miller School of Medicine, University of Miami Health System, University of Miami, Miami, FL, USA

Jackson Memorial Hospital, Jackson Health System, Miami, FL, USA
e-mail: ovelazquez@med.miami.edu

J. A. Freischlag
Wake Forest Baptist Health, Wake Forest School of Medicine, Winston-Salem, NC, USA
e-mail: jfreisch@wakehealth.edu

D. Farmer
Department of Surgery, UC Davis Children's Hospital, UC Davis Health System, UC Davis School of Medicine, Sacramento, CA, USA
e-mail: dlfarmer@ucdavis.edu

© Springer Nature Switzerland AG 2019
M. R. Kibbe, H. Chen (eds.), *Leadership in Surgery*, Success in Academic Surgery, https://doi.org/10.1007/978-3-030-19854-1_17

At Present

Women have made serious advances in the fields of medicine and surgery in the recent past, but 160 years after Elizabeth Blackwell's graduation from medical school, society is still far from gender parity. Although women now constitute roughly 50% of American medical students and enter academic medicine as faculty in numbers equal to their male colleagues, women are grossly underrepresented in positions of power and leadership [2, 3]. As of 2011, only 19% of tenured professors, 17% of full professors, 11.5% of department chairs, and 11% of deans (A total of 14 deans) were female [3]. If current trends continue, surgical resident will be equal proportions of men and women as early as the year 2028. The same trends, however, indicate that there will not be an equal number of male and female full professors of surgery until the year 2096 [4].

This leadership gap is not limited to medicine or surgery. It was long held that gender parity would be achieved as women entered the workforce in greater numbers. Referred to as the "pipeline effect," it was believed that women had not been present in sufficient numbers in the professional workforce for long enough to have advanced to senior leadership [3, 5, 6]. It was speculated that as more women entered the workforce they would move along the leadership pipeline, rise through the ranks and take a proportionate share of senior leadership roles. This has yet to happen, despite ample time. Although women have earned more than 50% of college degrees since the early 1980s, and currently outnumber men in management and professional occupations [3, 6], women make up only 16% of top executive positions in America's largest corporations. Only 17 countries in the world (out of 195) are led by women [6]. In the medical field, women are even underrepresented in leadership positions within the specialties dominated by women: for the past 25 years, 50% or more of psychiatrists, gynecologists and pediatricians have been female, and yet women constitute only 20% of full professors and 10% of department chairs within these specialties [3]. As Sheryl Sanberg wrote in Lean In—her Bestselling opus on female leadership—"The blunt truth is that men still rule the world" [6].

Even in a world run largely by men, surgery has long stood out as a particularly male dominated profession. The American College of Surgeons elected its first female chair to the board of regents in 2012, and no woman has ever served as the executive director. The American Surgical Association has only now (2015) elected a female president, and as of 2013 did not have any female council members. Of the eight regional surgical societies, three have never had a female president and an additional four have had only one [7]. Women in academic surgical departments are ten times more likely to perceive gender discrimination than their male colleagues. One study of 105 medical students indicated that 96% of female students viewed surgery as "unfavorable" to their gender [3]. Although by 2011 more than a third of general surgery residents were female, only 14% of full time faculty members were female. Faculty attrition remains substantial, with female surgeons at the assistant professor level being almost six times more likely to report an interest in leaving academia than male colleagues.

One study, conducted by Yedida and Bickel, conducted 80 min interviews with medical department chairs, and asked them to discuss the obstacles women face when rising through the ranks of academic medicine. The chairpersons identified three major barriers: traditional gender roles, sexism in the medical environment, and a lack of effective mentors [5].

Implicit Bias in Leadership

An often referenced study from Malcolm Gladwell's 2005 bestseller Blink finds that 30% of male CEOs from Fortune 500 companies are 6 ft 2 in. taller compared to 3.9% of Americans. This puts men of normal or below normal height at a disadvantage but it leaves the standing of women in leadership even lower. If leaders are supposed to be measured based off their values and accomplishments, why then is there such a blatant statistic showing otherwise? This is the notion of implicit bias— unconscious and unintentional control over one's perceptions [8]. Everyone, physicians included, are guilty of having implicit biases and the progressive of us seek to acknowledge and dismiss its influence.

Being uniquely tall does not translate to being an inherent leader. The genetics determining height or sex has no proven correlation between leadership efficacies. Rather, there exists an implicit bias that people prefer to "look-up", figuratively and practically, to taller male leaders. Perhaps this implicit bias formed over several generations of males in power identifying other males as the ideal leaders. Thankfully, our social atmosphere is rapidly changing but the looming projection of being decades away of true gender parity is debilitating. Women, without a doubt, are categorically underrepresented in leadership positions. A significant social shift needs to be made to address these concerns and acknowledge leadership ability on experience and capability rather than one's sex.

California, in an effort to address factors including systematic underrepresentation of women in leadership, became the first state to mandate that publically traded companies headquartered in California must have least one female director on its board [9]. This bold act will have a distinct effect on dozens of nationwide surgical-contracting companies and countless corporations.

Unfortunately, this does not disregard the rampant role that explicit bias plays, which is conscious and intentional bias, based on preconceived stereotypes. Through educational awareness and systematic reforms, the implicit and explicit bias that supports gender disparity is one step closer to being dismantled.

Leading from Any Seat: Julie Freischlag

When I was 7 years old, my grandfather shared words of wisdom that I still hold dear.

He said, "Julie, there are going to be people who say you can't do things in your life. When they say you can't, show them you can."

Although I didn't realize it at the time, my grandfather, who was a coal miner, was more than right. His advice to believe in myself has shaped my leadership experience as a woman in medicine—from my early days managing an operating room to my role today as CEO and Dean of a large learning health system.

In fact, being resilient, or "bouncing up" as I call it, is one of my mottos that has carried me through obstacles like implicit bias and gender discrimination. It has also given me the courage and inspiration to lead from any, and many, seats.

Early Days as "The Only"

My early days as a vascular surgeon and leader were filled with moments when I was "the only." I was the first woman faculty on staff at University of California at San Diego (UCSD) in 1987, and at University of California at Los Angeles (UCLA) in 1989. I was the second woman surgery faculty at the Medical College of Wisconsin and the only woman Vascular Surgery Division Chief in the country from 1998 to 2003.

One of my first direct experiences of gender stereotypes in surgery came as a young faculty member at University of California at San Diego (UCSD). My first case in the operating room was the placement of a Greenfield filter. I showed up early and sat quietly in the back of the room, where I overheard one of the nurses say, "The new vascular surgeon is doing this case. I wonder what he will be like." I knew the nurse had probably never worked with a woman faculty surgeon before, so the comment merely reflected the nurse's experience. She was quite surprised later to learn I was the surgeon on the case!

I also recall trying to find surgical gloves that fit my hands properly at the VA Hospital. The man in charge of the operating room responded to my request for 5½ size gloves, saying that he absolutely did not have that size. He only had size 6. After much discussion back and forth, size 5½ gloves were finally ordered. It turns out that many of the nurses had 5½ size hands too. Both of these experiences gave me an early peek into the implicit bias that women surgeons—and all women in medicine—often encounter, simply due to gender or size.

Dr. Caprice Greenberg, Professor of Surgery and Chair in Health Services Research at the University of Wisconsin, talked about the nature of implicit bias at the Annual Academic Surgical Congress Presidential Address. In her talk, called "Sticky Floors and Glass Ceilings," she said, "If you take away one lesson today, it is this: none of us are bad people, and none of us explicitly decide that men and women should be treated differently, but we all think this way—all of us. We all have implicit bias. Until we recognize this, embrace it, and identify the tools that we need to mitigate the impact of our biases, we are never going to be able to solve these problems" [10].

I believe she is correct, and even in my earliest days in the operating room, I didn't let the implicit bias I experienced hold me back. I continued being myself and bouncing ahead.

The Impostor Comes Calling

My first year out of training was tough—I questioned my abilities and felt like an impostor playing the role of surgeon. This was especially the case if one of my patient's suffered a complication or had an unfavorable outcome such as a wound or graft infection, thrombosed graft, stroke, bleeding or death.

Impostor Phenomenon was first described by Drs. Pauline R. Clance and Suzanne A. Imes in the article "The Impostor Phenomenon in High Achieving Women: Dynamics and Therapeutic Intervention" [11]. They described it as occurring most frequently in women, saying, "Despite outstanding academic and professional accomplishments, women who experience the impostor phenomenon persist in believing that they are really not bright and have fooled anyone who thinks otherwise [11]." While the definition was later expanded to include men, I think that feelings of inadequacy or not belonging can be particularly striking for women in surgery, due to the intense nature of the job and the fact that the field is male dominated.

During this time, I was fortunate to have two excellent young partners, Marc Sedwitz and Bob Hye, and a great Chief of Surgery at the VA, Bruce Stabile, as my mentors. Under their guidance, I developed a love of teaching and research that grew alongside my love of surgery. I conducted translational science research studying the role of neutrophils in reperfusion injury in both rat and rabbit hind limb ischemia models and acetylcholine-induced relaxation in arteries and veins from rabbits exposed to cigarette smoke and high cholesterol. I also became active in clinical trials as a principal investigator and led a research team, with students and residents working in my lab.

After 2 years in practice, I was offered a leadership position as Chief of Vascular Surgery at the West Los Angeles VA. For the next 6 years, I held many leadership roles, including Vice Chair of the Vascular Division at the Medical College of Wisconsin and Chief of Vascular Surgery at the Zablocki VA Medical Center in Milwaukee. I felt less and less like an impostor. It wasn't because of these leadership roles, though. It was because I had changed.

How? I believed in, and was inspired by, my many roles as surgeon, researcher, teacher, teammate and leader. My team of supporters had also broadened. In one instance at the Medical College of Wisconsin, my expertise was questioned. A senior male cardiologist asked my senior partner if I really knew what I was doing. My senior partner stood the ground with me. Shortly after that, a younger male anesthesiologist verbally assaulted and bullied me in the operating room, yelling about a case. This time, I stood up for myself and the issue was resolved. I had bounced up and was determined to stay there, without the impostor tagging along.

Leading Up, Down and Sideways

Being the Chief of Vascular Surgery at UCLA was an amazing opportunity to lead an entire team. It was there that I learned to lead in all directions—up, down, sideways and straight ahead. I wore many hats—clinical leader, surgeon, teacher, researcher and mentor. I took equal call as the rest of the division, operated every week and ran a translational science research lab studying carotid plaques in rabbits. Since almost everyone knew me because I trained there, implicit bias was practically non-existent and I could feel myself growing as a leader.

In this role, I led many who had trained me during residency, and this set of skills and relationships allowed me to develop influence in many directions. The one faculty member who initially wanted the job challenged me with some behaviors, such as saying he was not on call when he was and being quietly non-supportive. Over time, he became a loyal member of the division, and when I left after 5 years, he thanked me for my leadership. I think he realized that his strength was being a busy clinical vascular surgeon and teacher, and he saw the value of others leading administrative tasks and the division.

Additionally, I become part of a larger group who advised the Chair of Surgery. This taught me how all of the pieces fit together in a department. Once, the Chair of Surgery asked if I had only come to the meeting to make requests for vascular surgery. I, of course, said "Yes!" However, I soon learned that if I asked for my department plus others, the rewards would be quicker and larger. We were a team, after all! I was learning how to be an institutional leader.

Showing My True Colors

Dr. George Sheldon, who was going to retire as Chair of Surgery at University of North Carolina, was the first sponsor I had for a Chair of Surgery position. He put my name in for the position at the University of North Carolina, and even though I was not selected, my name was on the "list" for future chair positions. I interviewed at Southern Illinois University, Michigan State University, University of Colorado and University of Michigan. The fit either was not right from my point of view or theirs. One Dean even told me that I was a perfect fit, but the institution was not ready to hire a woman—they had no other women chairs. This was in 2002!

This all changed when I interviewed at Johns Hopkins. Dean Ed Miller embraced my vision to change the culture of surgery. The first 3 years at Johns Hopkins were the hardest of my career. I worked long hours, had a 7-year-old son and a husband who had moved for the second time across the country for my job.

The culture at Johns Hopkins was pretty cemented, and I was once again the lone woman among men. To begin the process of change, I hired many new surgeons, began new traditions and kept some of the old, while moving the department to new clinical, research and educational heights. Dean Miller was an amazing leader and an incredible sponsor.

I felt like an impostor multiple times. Since I was the only woman clinical chair for 11 years, I faced implicit bias as others questioned many of my actions. People even commented on my colorful clothes, so I wore black to blend in. Frustrated, I told the Senior Associate Dean of Faculty Affairs, Janice Clements, that I felt like I did not fit in. A very supportive leader, she encouraged me to carry on, because that is exactly why they hired me. They wanted someone different to lead!

After that, I wasn't afraid to show my true colors. One of my favorite photos from this time period shows the entire group of Johns Hopkins department chairs. I'm in a red silk jacket, and the rest of the chairs pictured are men in dark suits. I was no longer afraid to go above the fray of being watched and judged—I would lead. This definitely takes being brave and flexible and requires you to believe in yourself.

I also learned the three things I needed in my career to be a successful leader and feel fulfilled: a great boss, the opportunity to learn something new every day and the ability to make an impact. All of this came together during my time at Johns Hopkins and reflected in the many achievements our team made on a larger scale. Our research funding increased to the top 10 in surgery in the nation and philanthropy increased with eight lectureships and four professorships, with an annual amount of almost 10 million dollars per year. Our clinical activity increased every year, and we were present in five hospitals instead of two. I also operated throughout those years. In fact, during the first 5 years, I took call six to seven weekends per year and helped develop a top-notch thoracic outlet program and continued research as the national principal investigator on a VA clinical trial.

Still Bouncing

After Johns Hopkins, I decided I wanted to take the next step and be a Dean. In addition to being Chair of Surgery there, I also ran the operating room, where 550 surgical nurses reported to me, and I really enjoyed overseeing these operations. While I did not get the job at Johns Hopkins, I became a Dean and Vice Chancellor at UC Davis. During this job search, which included job interviews at two other institutions, I experienced implicit bias. Many thought a surgeon could not oversee more than surgery and that surgeons were poor listeners who made decisions only to benefit themselves. I felt qualified for the position and far from this description. The impostor did not come calling this time! I did however realize I needed to do some convincing that I was a surgeon who could lead in a harmonious, team-oriented way.

My boss at UC Davis was Chancellor Linda Katehi, who was an electrical engineer and originated from Greece. She taught me so much about leading as a woman in her position. She had a different style of leadership which was inclusive and very outside the box. The previous Dean and Vice Chancellor was a woman, so I felt very little implicit bias. I did have a steep learning curve however as I had not been involved in undergraduate, medical student and resident education outside of surgery. My first year was focused on getting up to speed in those arenas. I knew that the key to larger scope jobs is getting the right team together and creating a vision and strategic direction together.

I also started a symposia series in each department and center where junior faculty presented research. These were very well received and exciting. Our research funding increased by 5–10% every year, and we used many of the research ideas to lead fundraising asks. As a result, our fundraising total doubled in 2 years. During this time, I also continued to do clinical trials research, operated about twice each month and started a thoracic outlet program with my younger partner Misty Humphries.

Yes, I Can!

Where has my journey brought me? I am now CEO and Dean at Wake Forest Baptist Health in Winston-Salem, North Carolina. There is great deal of diversity, innovation and expertise here. I am no longer "the only" and am surrounded by an amazing group of women leaders and surgeons.

The culture is very collaborative. People are ready for changes, and we are making them. I have actually felt no implicit bias due to my skill set and leadership ability. I have had a bit of impostor syndrome as we are doing a few things I have not done in the past, like mergers and acquisitions, balancing a tough budget due to lack of Medicaid expansion, and replacing a few chairs in the first year. However, I don't experience impostor syndrome in the same way I did early in my career, because I have the right people on my team and trust myself as a leader.

If those old feelings do start to return, I keep in mind a few tips that Dr. Sharon Hull, Director of the Duke University School of Medicine Executive Coaching Program and Professor, Community and Family Medicine, gave when she presented at a women's leadership conference at Wake Forest Baptist. She referred to impostor syndrome as "the gnome on your shoulder" and shared four tips on how to "quiet the gnome." She advised: "recognize that impostor syndrome is real and common; talk with others whom you trust about your experience; recognize that when the gnome shows up, it is a signal that you're in a stretch period and need to build some skills; and bring some humor to the problem—dance with your gnome!" [12].

I hold onto this advice and also focus on areas where I feel confident in my expertise, like surgery and research, while learning leadership roles that are new to me. I continue to see thoracic outlet patients and operate about twice each month with my younger partner Gabriela Velazquez. I'm also active in research and recently presented the 10-year follow up for the VA clinical trial at the American College of Surgeons meeting.

As the leader of this large organization, I know that culture does control the extent of one's success, and that every interaction adds up to so much more. Therefore, it is important to spend time getting to know the culture and the people who make your organization unique. Almost 20,000 people work at Wake Forest Baptist. I connect face-to-face, hold town halls across the health system, touch base with every department, and use other types of messaging like monthly videos and social media. I walk the halls and show up for as many events as I can at the Medical Center. I get joy out of participating in community activities and chaired the March of Dimes and American Heart & Stroke Walk this past year.

I've seen firsthand the power of connections in leadership, through mentorship and sponsorship, and in the people I work with every day. I've also seen how the advice my grandfather gave me years ago to be brave, bounce up and believe in myself—and others—still rings true today.

Remember, "When they say you can't, show them you can." You CAN lead from any seat!

Adaptability Overcomes Adversity: An Improbable Journey of Surreal Proportions—Omaida C. Velazquez

The number of women enrolling in US medical schools currently exceeds the number of men and they achieve graduation in the top quartile of their class similarly to men. Yet, since the Halsted introduction of a formalized system in which medical school graduates enter a university-sponsored, hospital-based surgical training program [13], we have to still envision a formalized plan to ensure that future surgical talent is gathered from a gender-diverse pool reflective of modern-day medical school's graduating classes. How do we create such pool? Clearly the onus is on us, our profession's leaders. As surgical leaders, we must heed the calling to cultivate and attract the top medical students into that prospective pool and to forge leaders among our diverse members. To do that effectively, we need to be proactive and goal-directed, aiming to reduce the significant under-representation of women choosing our field and serving as leaders in our field. By sharing my story, the goal is to illuminate the behind the scenes destructive and constructive forces at play in a woman's path to leadership in American Surgery.

My path has taken me to become a leader, mentor, sponsor and role model. As the first Latina Chair and Surgeon-in-Chief in America, I've embraced the concept that strong leadership should encompass all the above. That I would come to serve in this capacity, did not ever seem feasible and was certainly not planned, but perhaps my unconventional path prepared me for these leadership roles. It was a rocky path with many challenges along the way. Throughout it all my own mentors, sponsors, and role models along with a healthy dose of adaptability were instrumental in making it possible. I draw from my life experiences to be an effective leader, a collaborator, and an advocate for patients, learners, and faculty. My story illustrates that women and minorities can lead effectively and bring a unique perspective that can complement and enrich any leadership team.

Childhood

Born and raised in Pinar Del Rio, Cuba, there was a time as a child, when the basic modern amenities that we now take for granted (electricity, running water, indoor plumbing, and basic freedoms) were not accessible. Determined not to dwell on things impossible to change, I adapted and pushed ahead with a dream for better days. Although books and magazines were scarce, reading every available page on every subject became my quest. It was in early childhood that I first encounter inequities across genders and discriminatory practices based on the color of people's skin or their religion. Unhappy with the conditions, I dreamed what seemed impossible, leave my beautiful island of Cuba and scape to America. When the dream miraculously came to pass, survival and success would've not been possible without extraordinary adaptability and great mentors, sponsors, and role models along the way. The resilience skills from my early years were the foundation for overcoming many obstacles to come, many destructive forces.

By the age of 14 I had moved over a half dozen times in my parent's endless pursuit of a better life and freedom. Born in a rural and remote area, the most trans-formational relocation brought me to Union City, New Jersey. As a child, I had often day dreamed of traveling to the USA, it seemed so improbable that I had filed it away in my mental shelf of fantasies. One unforgettable afternoon, I left early from school at the request of my parents. When I arrived home, my mom and dad were packing. I didn't know it then, but we were about to join the 1980 Mariel Boatlift, sponsored by our family who had migrated to the US in the early 1960s. That day was to show me the best and worst of the human nature.

After surviving the mobs intended on lethal harm for the crime of leaving the island, we endured a week of unsheltered, concentration camp-like treatment at the port of Mariel (west of Habana) before finally boarding a boat full of dissidents under the moonlight and with a storm approaching. A journey that was supposed to be only a couple of hours lasted all night and then some. When our small boat finally arrived at Key West, Florida, filled to the brim with exiles, Spanish-speaking volun-teers received us with Coca Cola and M&Ms. To a dehydrated, nauseous 14-year-old girl, it was like arriving in heaven and being received by angels.

Later, while flying to Fort Chaffee, Arkansas, the elated feelings would rapidly vanish, replaced by a foreboding out-of-body experience that lasted the entire month there. It felt like being inside one of those old sub-titled black-and-white movies I had once seen as a child (but without the subtitles). For many years, every experi-ence in America felt surreal, even the escalators, the revolving doors, and trips to the supermarkets. The stigma associated with the Mariel immigrants stuck with me, always pulling me down. Although I was offered political asylum and became an American citizen, many continued to view me as a "marielita" (an invisible destruc-tive, marginalizing force).

Education in America

A leader among American high school teachers, Nadia Makar, was my first mentor, at Union Hill High School, in Union City, NJ. She recognized something in me that I knew was there, but all others didn't. Since my arrival to the US, I expressed my goal of pursuing a career in Medicine. But, the idea of acceptance into medical school in America, not speaking English at age 14 and coming from an inner city high school seem ludicrous. There were no shortage of people pointing out the obvi-ous impossibility and naiveté of the mere concept. But all I needed was one sup-porter and the willingness to adopt to anything (working in a dry cleaning store in New York City, being constantly undervalued and underestimated at first glance, and being treated as 'forever a girl'). Walking the streets of Union City, I endured the embarrassment of whistling and inappropriate sexually charged remarks from chauvinistic boys and men. Over many years since my arrival from Cuba, I was painfully reserved. I almost never smiled and rarely volunteered to speak. My grandmother, Julia, always prompted me, "sonriete", "habla tu mente" translating to "smile" and "speak your mind".

In high school, students and even my designated high school guidance counselor tried to convince me that my background made it impossible to get into any competitive college. Later, in college, at Stevens Institute of Technology, a chemistry professor invited me to his office to advise me that Medicine was a very bad career choice for "girls" because I would never experience the joy of getting married, having a family or becoming a mother. In medical school, several colleagues and professors advised against Surgery as a career because "it was too hard" and I "I was too nice" and "a bit petite for surgery that is very physical". Another common deterrence line was "most female surgeons can't find the time to have children." Interestingly, I never refuted or openly tussled against such biases. And a part of me internalized the misguided remarks. Even as a surgical division chief, a colleague of mine once said, "naturally you have that 'respect of the male figure' ingrained as part of your Cuban culture, so it may be hard for you". I said nothing in response. The reality was that every one of these individuals (despite their biases) are intrinsically good people, and genuinely believe that they are providing good advice. Implicit bias is like that, always hidden deep within our consciousness.

My approach was to keep an ever positive frame of mind, I studied, engaged, participated and followed an unwavering path from high school to college to a full merit-scholarship at University of Medicine and Dentistry of New Jersey—New Jersey Medical School (UMDNJ-NJMS); now Rutgers University-NJMS. I would ultimately graduate Valedictorian in my medical school class of 1991, 11 years after my improbable and surreal journey to America. Mentors, sponsors, role-models, and advisors made all the difference in my career. In medical school, renowned biochemist Dr. Michael Lea taught me the love of biomedical research. He inspired me to see research as the most impactful way to contribute to future generations. Trauma surgeon, Kenneth Swan extended that research passion into the idea that surgeons had been responsible for discovering many cures and that the academic surgeon was essential to continue the chain of critical discoveries within Medicine. His dedication and passion to clinical surgery and to discovery were infectious. When I shared my interest in surgery with him, my gender never came up; it was a non-issue. His sponsorship and that of Dr. Benjamin Rush (chair of surgery for 25 years at UMDNJ-NJMS) were instrumental in my acceptance to the Hospital of the University of Pennsylvania (HUP) as a categorical resident in General Surgery.

Dr. Clyde Barker was my first chair of Surgery at HUP and after graduating from the General Surgery program there, Clyde and the Vascular Surgery faculty selected me as their first female Vascular Surgery Fellow. Upon completion of my fellowship Clyde offered me a job on the tenure-earning track and I became the first woman on the Vascular Surgery Faculty at HUP. Many years later, when I was inducted to the American Society of Clinical Investigators (ASCI), Clyde sent me a wonderful hand-written congratulatory letter (I was by then in Miami, as chief of the vascular division). Clyde was the chair during my training and first 4 years as a faculty member at HUP. Like Nadia, he believed in me when he took me into his categorical residency class and when he hired me in the Tenure earning track. In the subsequent 4 years, Larry Kaiser (who succeeded Clyde Barker as my next chair of surgery), also offered strong support and sponsorship. While at HUP, great role models and mentors such as Ronald Fairman, Michael Golden and Jeff Carpenter were my teachers in the art of clinical vascular and endovascular surgery and it was great to spend 8 years with them as their colleague faculty member.

At HUP, accomplished women leaders in American Surgery, Jo Buyske and Kim Olthoff, were great role models. I observed and admired the way in which they seamlessly integrated their roles as mother and surgeon. And how they took leadership roles with dedication and great competency. As a PGY3, 1 year before my formal 2 years of research training, I took the plunge into motherhood. Having a pregnant PGY3 resident was 'a first' in the history of the HUP surgery training program. It was such a big deal that I announced in a private meeting with Clyde; he was the second to know after my husband. But, Clyde Barker, Bill Schwab, and by the most part, all the training faculty were either unperturbed or well versed at not showing it. In any event, my pregnancy was uneventful and thereafter many women surgical trainees did not hesitate to routinely start their family during training. My first born child came 2 weeks into my 2-year research lab experience. Those years were the most significant towards my maturation as a surgeon scientist.

My mentor, Dr. John Rombeau, not only trained me ('Halsted style') as a meticulous clinical surgeon, but also taught me the scientific principles and reinforced my early love for discovery such that it became completely embedded and integrated in my holistic view of academic surgery. From those seminal years came a philosophy that I adopted from John Rombeau; *as surgeon one can help a patient at a time in the present but as a surgeon scientist one could help countless millions in the future*. He also often related his advice to young surgeon-scientists that *the key to perseverance in research is to never allow yourself 'to get too high or too low'*. He is indeed the quintessential mentor whose philosophy and passion for surgical mentorship is beautifully captured in his book *Surgical Mentoring: Building Tomorrow's Leaders* [14].

Considering Leadership Roles

In Philadelphia, I gained clinical skills in both adult and pediatric vascular surgery. In Pediatric vascular, I ultimately became the go-to surgeon at the Children's Hospital of Philadelphia (CHOP). This skill plus adult advanced open and endovascular clinical experience together with my funded research was being noticed nationally and resulted in some invitations for looking at leadership positions. Eight years into my service at HUP/CHOP, I became tenured at the University of Pennsylvania, at the Associate Professor level. During those years, I remember Julie Freischlag once shared with me that when she hires a leader, she first considers their performance in prior formative leadership roles. Julie has been an advisor and role model for me and many women in academic surgery. Shortly after that conversation I became receptive to the idea of evaluating leadership opportunities. In 2007, I was recruited to the University of Miami Miller School of Medicine and UHealth System as Chief of the Division of Vascular and Endovascular Surgery. Over subsequent years at University of Miami, I've assumed several leadership roles, such Vice Chair for Research in the Department of Surgery and Executive Dean for Research in the medical school, ultimately accepting my current position as chair and surgeon-in-chief.

Craig Kent, who over the years has been a role model and advisor suggested to start looking at chair positions, about 6 months before my chair in Miami, Alan Livingstone decided to step down. So by the time the Miami chair position was open and under national search, I was already under serious consideration in the active searches for two other possible chair jobs. Ultimately, I was offered the Miami position which was in my mind a great fit for me and the institution. My first Dean at the Miller School of Medicine, Pascal Goldschmidt was a tremendous mentor, role model, and sponsor since my arrival at the University of Miami. Our president at the time, Donna Shalala, was also a great supporter of my career and became a sponsor as well as one of my most influential role models.

Attracting superstars, supporting women and underrepresented minorities, advancing the careers of my faculty and building clinical programs has been the focus of my leadership roles in Miami. Along the way, research from my Lab on vascular biology, angiogenesis, atherosclerosis, and diabetic wound healing was NIH-funded in Philadelphia and remains so, to date. Work from my Lab has yielded several patents and most recently a new pre-clinical treatment with translational promise for peripheral vascular disease, recognized by the NIH and my current institution and now housed within a new start-up company. Our UM department of Surgery's education programs have prospered, with new vascular independent and integrated training programs initiated and with the core general surgery program matching seven categorical spots from the top 11 ranked in the 2017 entry class. Currently, under our new leadership at UM, Dean Henri Ford, CEO, Ed Abraham, Provost Jeffrey Duerk and President Julio Frenk, the department of Surgery continues to have strong support and fostering gender-diversity continues to be at the forefront of our institutional priorities.

As is the case for many women in medicine, given the relative paucity of women at the top of leadership and influence, the majority of my mentors and sponsors are men. I think of them as enlighten leaders who adopted the cause of diversity and inclusiveness way before it was a popularized concept; and they are able to suspend the natural human implicit biases and recognize talent, regardless of gender. As to my women mentors, advisors, and role-models—without them, my path to leadership and academic contributions would not have even started. Most humbling to me, is that over time, I have become a mentor, sponsor and role-model with many mentees whose successes make us all proud. One such superstar mentee is Kathy Gallagher, an accomplished, NIH-funded surgeon scientist [15]. This year, another one of my highly talented mentees, surgeon-in-training Dr. Punam P. Parikh humbled me with a beautifully and elegantly written chapter on surgical mentorship where she candidly describes our mentor-mentee experience [16]:

Frankly, I aspired to emulate her both personally and professionally. The origins of this mentor-mentee relationship started even earlier in my career path (when I was a medical student)

Many women leaders have a servant-leader approach and seek talent with a conscious and proactive priority of increasing diversity. This is perhaps easier for women because they've experienced gender bias and have been able to adapt, succeed and turn the bad experiences into an impetus to eliminate discrimination.

Time to Change

In the book, *The Order Of Time* by Carlo Rovelli, an Italian Theoretical Physicist, he elegantly explains that based on our latest understanding, there is no such thing as a universal 'present', nor an absolute 'here and now':

Our "present" does not extend throughout the universe. It is like a bubble around us [17].

There is no absolute 'present' in the fundamental fabric of our world, only the experiences of the past that shape what will become of us in the future. There is a marvelous sense of revelation when leaving the microelements of the daily routine and zooming out to glimpse the surprising elemental reality of our physical world. Indeed, my "present" has always seemed a surreal, improbable state, materialized from a rapidly changing past and a fantastical and improvable envisioned future. Such tumultuous journey can only be endured by the special savvy of 'adaptability' and with great counsel. There has never been a time where sudden changes and adversity was not part and center of my personal and professional path. Yet, it always seemed easy to keep grip on the bumpy road through mindful adaptation and willingness to listen to good advice.

Rovelli goes on to explain, "The entire evolution of science would suggest that the best grammar for thinking about the world is that of change, not of permanence. Not of being, but of becoming" [17].

Therefore, change in our field is not an option but a predestined reality. The question is can we frame the direction and nature of the change aiming to eliminate implicit bias and create equitable gender representation. Women leaders intuitively, through self-experience and heighten sense of empathy, lead in the spirit of these principles and goals. And they bring that essential perspective to the table of individuals influencing and crafting the changing faces of leadership in Surgery.

In Summary

At the time of this writing there are 22 women Chairs of Surgery in the United States. Clearly progress has been made. But sadly, the bias that women surgeons encounter in their day to day roles remains.

Women who are demanding of excellence in the operating rooms and clinics are more often labeled "bitches" and more frequently accused of creating a hostile environment. Men need to cuss, use foul language or throw things before they are "written up" whereas for women the discrimination is more insidious and passive aggressive.

Whether having women surgeons in the operating room upsets the long established (read white straight male dominated) status quo or whether it is a problem with women leading other women and men in support roles; the root causes may be different but the outcome remains the same—women and minorities still need to "be better" to get ahead and achieve parity.

It has been 40 years since the Equal Rights Amendment failed to pass. How odd that someone opposes that "Equality of rights under the law shall not be denied or abridged by the United States or by any state on account of sex." We cannot give up the fight for ourselves and for our patients. Women must continue to lead, to seek leadership positions, and hire more women and underrepresented minorities. The resistance will get greater as the majority sees the inevitable historical power base recede. We need to do this for our children, for health care, and for the health of the planet.

Acknowledgments *We acknowledge and thank Julian Costa, Katherine Files and Gelsys Sargenton for their outstanding assistance with coordinating, organizing and compiling the completed manuscript.*

References

1. Gartzia L, Van Engen M. Are (male) leaders "feminine" enough? Gendered traits of identity as mediators of sex differences in leadership styles. Gend Manag Int J. 2012;27(5):296–314.
2. McLemore EC, et al. Women in surgery: bright, sharp, brave, and temperate. Perm J. 2012;16(3):54–9.
3. Lillemoe KD, Ahrendt GM, Yeo CJ, Herlong HF, Cameron JL. Surgery – still an "old boys' club"? Surgery. 1994;116(2):255–9.
4. Sexton KW, et al. Women in academic surgery: the pipeline is busted. J Surg Educ. 2012;69(1):84–90.
5. Yedidia MJ, Bickel J. Why aren't there more women leaders in academic medicine? The views of clinical department chairs. Acad Med. 2001;76(5):453–65.
6. Sandberg S. Lean in. New York, NY: Alfred A Knopf; 2013.
7. Cochran A, Freischlag J, Numann P. Women, surgery, and leadership: where we have been, where we are, where we are going. JAMA Surg. 2013;148(4):312–3.
8. Greenwald AG, Krieger LH. Implicit bias: scientific foundations. Calif Law Rev. 2006;94(4):945–67.
9. Fuhrmans V, Lazo A. California moves to mandate female board directors. Wall Street J. 29 Aug, 2018. https://www.wsj.com/articles/california-moves-to-mandate-female-board-directors-1535571904?mod=article_inline.
10. Greenberg CC. Association for Academic Surgery presidential address: sticky floors and glass ceilings. J Surg Res. 2017;219:ix–xviii.
11. Clance PR, Imes SA. The impostor phenomenon in high achieving women: dynamics and therapeutic intervention. Psychother Theor Res Pract. 1978;15(3):241–7.

12. Hull SK. The impostor syndrome: dancing with the gnome on your shoulder. In: Presentation at Women's Leadership Conference, Breakthrough to Brave, Wake Forest Baptist Medical Center, Fall; 2018.
13. Halsted WS. The training of the surgeon. Bull Johns Hopkins Hosp. 1904;xv:267–75.
14. Rombeau JL, Goldberg A, Loveland-Jones C. Surgical mentoring: building tomorrow's leaders. Berlin: Springer Science+Business Media, LLC; 2010.
15. Gallagher K. Spotlight on leadership: interview with Omaida Velazquez, MD. Soc Vasc Surg Vasc Spec. 2018;14(1):15–6.
16. Parikh P, Lew L, Velazquez OC. The importance of leadership and mentorship in surgery: an anecdotal account and philosophical construct. In: …43rd Annual Northwester Vascular Symposium; 2018.
17. Rovelli C. The order of time. New York, NY: Riverhead Books/Penguin Random House LLC; 2018.

What Does It Mean to Be an Underrepresented Minority Leader in Surgery

18

Jeffrey S. Upperman, Jessica N. Rea, and Henri R. Ford

Introduction

A culturally diverse work force is important in addressing health disparities [1–5]. Yet underrepresented minority in medicine physicians (URMM) remain relatively scarce in the health care work force. In fact, African-, Hispanic-, and Native-Americans in particular are underrepresented in surgery—especially academic surgery. This disparity is due to multifactorial reasons and the main reason is a dearth of URMM candidates in the pipeline. In other words, the gap between the proportion of the U.S. minority population and the percentage of these students graduating from U.S. medical schools continues to widen. As a consequence, URMM surgical leaders, who have made it through the gauntlet of the complex climb from pre-medical training to the politics of faculty life in academic health centers, face responsibilities as URMM surgical leaders that their counterparts may not encounter. For instance, they not only must establish their legitimacy as academic superstars and earn the respect and esteem of the broader surgical community, but also serve as URMM role models, advocates, mentors and sponsors for surgical trainees and faculty, and finally, as social activists for reducing or eliminating health disparities. In this chapter, these themes are explored in the context of academic surgery,

J. S. Upperman (✉)
Department of Surgery, Keck School of Medicine of the University of Southern California, Los Angeles, CA, USA

Children's Hospital Los Angeles, Los Angeles, CA, USA
e-mail: JUpperman@chla.usc.edu

J. N. Rea
Children's Hospital Los Angeles, Los Angeles, CA, USA

H. R. Ford
Millier School of Medicine, Miami, FI, USA
e-mail: hford@med.miami.edu

© Springer Nature Switzerland AG 2019
M. R. Kibbe, H. Chen (eds.), *Leadership in Surgery*, Success in Academic Surgery, https://doi.org/10.1007/978-3-030-19854-1_18

and we will present the approach to overcoming some of these barriers by illustrating the work of pioneering URMM surgical leaders.

Barriers to Attaining a Position of Leadership in Academic Surgery

Health disparities between the minority populations and European-Americans remain a vexing problem in contemporary American society. Minorities have shorter life expectancies and suffer a disproportionately higher rate of cardiovascular disease, cancer, birth defects, asthma, diabetes, stroke, sexually transmitted diseases and mental illness than whites [1, 2]. The etiology of such disparities is multifactorial with historical implications and includes, but is not limited to, inequalities in income and education, biological differences among ethnic groups, cultural dissonance, access to and quality of health care, as well as racial and ethnic discrimination. In fact, the Institute of Medicine argues that racial or ethnic prejudice on the part of health care providers underlies disparities in health care for URMM even when they have adequate or equal access [1]. Thus, a culturally diverse work force is important for addressing health disparities. Given the fact that physicians from URMM are more likely to practice in underserved areas following completion of their training, regardless of their chosen subspecialty, this argument provides greater impetus to train more URMM physicians in an effort to mitigate the effects of racial and ethnic discrimination [4]. Yet URMM physicians remain markedly underrepresented in the medical work force, and there are small numbers of African-, Hispanic-, and Native-Americans in academic surgery.

To understand the dearth of African-, Hispanic-, and Native-Americans in academic surgery, one needs to consider the decrease in candidates along the academic pipeline. Although African-, Hispanic-, and Native-Americans comprised 33% of the United States population in 2017 combined, they accounted for only 12% of U.S. medical students that same year [6, 7] (Table 18.1). In 2017, these URMMs accounted for less than 13% of surgical residents in the U.S. [9]. Among U.S. surgical faculty, URMMs accounted for only 6% and roughly 3% of the tenured surgical faculty [8]. Thus, given the small pool of surgical residents, it is understandable that there are a disproportionately lower number of URMM physicians on the surgical faculty at most institutions, and consequently in leadership positions in academic surgery.

In spite of increasing numbers of medical students graduating from U.S. medical schools over the past 5 years, there remains a disparity between URMM medical school graduates and the relative population proportion in the U.S. For instance, in 2013, African-, Hispanic-, and Native-Americans accounted for 10% of U.S. medical school graduates and 31% of the U.S. population [3, 10]. By 2018, there was a net increase of 1099 medical school graduates during that 5-year period. European-American students accounted for 5%, Asian-Americans for 37%, while African-, Hispanic-, and Native-Americans accounted for 7%, 10%, and 0.6% of the net increase respectively. Overall, URMMs accounted for 11% of U.S. medical school graduates in 2018 while representing 33% of the U.S. population [11]. Thus, despite the overall increase in the number of medical school graduates, the gap between the

Table 18.1 Profile of U.S. population and medical school matriculants

	2017 U.S. population [6]	2017–2018 U.S. medical school matriculants [7]	2017 U.S. surgical residents[a] [9]	2017 U.S. surgical faculty[a] [8]	2017 U.S. surgical tenured professors[a] [8]
European-American	60.7%	52%	69.2%	62.5%	77.9%
African-American	13.4%	5.6%	4.8%	3.5%	1.4%
Asian-American	5.8%	21.4%	18.7%	18.3%	8.0%
Hispanic-American	18.1%	6.4%	7.2%	2.2%	1.6%
Native-American	1.3%	0.23%	0.22%	0.2%	0.01%
Pacific-Islander	0.2%	0.1%	UD[b]	0.06%	0.01%
≥2 races	2.7%	UD[b]	UD[b]	8.4%	6.4%
Non-U.S. Citizen and Non-Permanent Residents	UD[b]	1.51%	UD[b]	UD[b]	UD[b]
Other	UD[b]	UD[b]	UD[b]	5.1%	3.5%

[a]General surgery
[b]*UD* undefined

proportion of the U.S. population of URMMs and the populations graduating from U.S. medical schools persists. This trend is particularly concerning since Hispanic-Americans and African-Americans will grow to nearly 35% of the U.S. population by the year 2030. Beyond that, by the year 2020, African-Americans and Hispanic-Americans will account for over 37% of the college age population (18 year-olds), which represents the future pool of U.S. physicians [12]. Failure to understand and reverse this alarming trend could result in increasing health care disparities.

The foregoing paragraphs suggest that one of the key barriers to having more URMM surgeons assuming leadership positions in academic surgery is the relatively small pool of candidates in the pipeline. For those URMM students who aspire to pursue a surgical career after graduating from medical school, they face challenges during surgical residency and as junior faculty that may impede their professional development and subsequent advancement up the academic ladder (Fig. 18.1). Challenges include lack of URMM role models and mentors, insufficient counseling, minimal financial support and research infrastructure [5, 12–14]. Many of these barriers are not specific to URMMs but they can be amplified if the URMM lacks the social capital to overcome these barriers at a particular institution.

Trailblazers in Overcoming These Barriers

Trailblazers such as Charles Drew and Samuel L. Kountz, and more recently, LaSalle Leffall, Claude Organ, and L.D. Britt, to name a few, have been able to overcome all sorts of barriers to reach the apogee of American Surgery. These giants of American surgery, who happen to be from an URMM, share one common thread: they personified excellence. According to an anonymous writer, excellence is the "the result of caring more than others think is wise, risking more than others think is safe, dreaming more than others think is practical, and

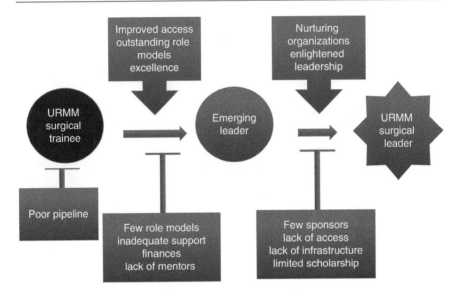

Fig. 18.1 Barriers that impede professional advancement of potential URMM leaders along the academic ladder and potential remedies

expecting more than others think is possible." Indeed, these pioneers exemplified the notion that excellence will silence all critics. Undoubtedly, they would be inducted into the "Hall of Fame of American Surgery" if such an entity existed. The following paragraphs will highlight some of the phenomenal URMMs in American surgery and serve as examples of outstanding results that are possible against all odds.

Daniel Hale Williams served as Vice President of the National Medical Association and was the only African-American charter member of the American College of Surgeons. Credited with performing the first successful open heart surgery after carefully asserting no other surgeon completed such feat in 1893, Williams also established a lasting legacy by founding the first non-segregated hospital in the U.S.: Chicago's Provident Hospital [15]. During his service as Chief of Surgery at Freedmen's Hospital, he welcomed the community to come scrutinize, criticize, and attempt find flaw in the technique of African-American surgeons in order to demonstrate the capabilities of their skill [16].

Having served at Howard University/Freedman's Hospital as faculty to improve the education of African-American surgeons, Charles R. Drew epitomized excellence. His brilliant work while a research fellow and surgery resident at Columbia University Presbyterian Hospital helped to elucidate the causative factors in the pathogenesis of shock. In conjunction with John Scudder, he studied the efficacy of blood plasma in the treatment of secondary shock. It is widely held that his doctoral thesis on "Banked Blood" not only provided the basis for separating the components of whole blood, such as plasma from the red cells, but also may have led to the establishment of the modern blood bank [17]. As such, he was appointed Director of the first American Red Cross Blood Bank at Presbyterian Hospital. Not only does Charles Drew's legacy include his innovations in blood banking, it also encompasses the training and mentorship of such surgeons as Asa Yancey, LaSalle Leffall, William Sinkler, and many more.

Asa Yancey Jr. was the eighth resident at Freedman's Hospital, training under Charles Drew [18]. Asa Yancey's excellence in surgery would later translate to an important advancement in the management of Hirschsprung's Disease. He first reported on the modification of the Swenson technique in the Journal of the National Medical Association in 1952 [19]. Despite his publication, Soave is credited with the modification [18].

Similarly, Samuel L. Kountz distinguished himself as a superb academic surgeon. His seminal work on the "Mechanism of Rejection of Homotransplanted Kidneys" was published in *Nature* in 1963 [17]. In addition to serving as Chair of the Department of Surgery at the State University of New York at Downstate, he held numerous leadership positions in prestigious academic surgical societies, ultimately culminating with his ascendancy to the Presidency of the Society of University Surgeons in 1975. Samuel L. Kountz later erected the Center for Human Values at UCSF to discuss ethical issues about transplants with an overall goal to improve the care of African-Americans in urban areas [20].

Dorothy Lavinia Brown is said to have declared, "Dr. Matthew Walker was a brave man" of Matthew Walker who accepted her into Meharry's surgical residency [21]. She was the first African-American woman to become a Fellow of the ACS, and the first African-American woman senate in the state of Tennessee in 1966. Women's health care and livelihood were her passion, and she believed that a bill regarding abortion rights would have the potential of saving many Tennessee women [21]. Unfortunately, the bill did not pass. Beyond the awards and buildings named after Dr. Brown, she was a role model in every meaning of the phrase [21].

The first URMM President of the American College of Surgeons was LaSalle D. Leffall, Jr. Dr. Leffall's brilliance was evident as early as his high school years, when he was named valedictorian of his class at 15 years old [22]. He repeated this feat 7 years later at Howard University College of Medicine, graduating at the top of his class. This was followed by a fellowship in surgical oncology at Memorial Sloan Kettering Hospital during which he distinguished himself as one of the stellar fellows. Upon his return as an Assistant Professor of Surgery at Howard University, he quickly rose through the ranks to become Chair of the Department. In addition, as a distinguished surgical oncologist, he rose to become President of the American Cancer Society and the Society of Surgical Oncology, the first African-American to hold these positions, prior to his election as President of the American College of Surgeons in 1995. Finally, in 2002, he was named chairman of the President's Cancer Panel.

Claude H. Organ, Jr. holds the distinction of being the first African-American to assume the Chairmanship of a Department of Surgery at a predominantly white medical school, his alma mater, Creighton University [23]. His tremendous work ethic, exceptional commitment to excellence, and unparalleled dedication to mentoring not only earned him the respect of his colleagues and students but also contributed to his success as an academic surgeon. Dr. Organ was the first African-American editor of the surgical journal with the largest distribution in the country, Archives of Surgery. His two-volume historical text on African-American surgeons remains an invaluable addition to his legacy [24]. In addition, he was a founding member of the Society of Black Academic Surgeons, an organization devoted to promoting mentoring and scholarship among surgical trainees and faculty from an URMM background. In 2003, Dr. Organ became the second African-American President of the American College of Surgeons.

L.D. Britt graduated from Harvard Medical School and Harvard School of Public Health on his way to becoming the first African-American Professor of Surgery in the Commonwealth of Virginia and chair of the department of surgery at Eastern Virginia Medical School [25]. During his tenure, he has received numerous accolades nationally and internationally, including the Robert J. Glaser Distinguished Educator Award, the highest teaching award or accolade in medicine given by the Association of American Medical Colleges [26]. He has served as President of numerous prestigious academic surgical societies including the Southern Surgical Society, the American Surgical Association, the American Association for the Surgery of Trauma, the Society of Black Academic Surgeons, and the American College of Surgeons.

In 1994, Lori Arviso Alvord became the first Navajo woman board certified in surgery. She bridges traditional Navajo healing and Western medicine to treat her patients. Her appointments in leadership have led her to serve as Associate Dean for Student Affairs at Dartmouth Medical School (1997–2009), and, more recently, associate dean for student affairs and admissions at the University of Arizona College of Medicine in Tucson (2012–present) [27]. Throughout her academic appointments, Lori Arviso Alvord emphasized elements of her Navajo culture into her practice. It is a long time coming for Native American representation.

Likewise, Alfredo Quiñones-Hinojosa is a neurosurgeon who crossed the U.S.-Mexico border for the purpose of a better life. He worked as a migrant worker, eventually leaving this job at the advice of his cousin [28]. Alfredo Quiñones-Hinojosa's work ethic and excellence in performance certainly transcended the barrier of immigration in the U.S. Certainly, there is a national divide with the repeal of the Development, Relief, and Education for alien Minors Act (DREAM) Act and, more recently, President Barack Obama's Deferred Action for Childhood Arrivals (DACA) program. And with the ongoing health disparity and URMM crises, this nation needs giants like Alfredo Quiñones-Hinojosa.

There are many other worthy URMM surgical leaders who have had to overcome significant barriers to ultimately play an influential role in American surgery. Suffice it to say, they all shared the same relentless passion for the pursuit of excellence. However, while one can argue that excellence is the essential scaffold for success, it is the quest for significance, or the desire to make the biggest difference possible in the lives of others and in their community, that propelled these trailblazers, legendary pioneers and role models to the heights of American surgery.

What Are the Challenges Facing Surgical Leader from an URMM?

"True leadership lies in guiding others to success. In ensuring that everyone is performing at their best, doing the work they are pledged to do and doing it well."—Bill Owens

"The growth and development of people is the highest calling of leadership."—Harvey Firestone

One of the challenging problems that impede the development of surgical leaders from an URMM is the vicious cycle fueled by a limited pipeline, lack of diversity in the surgical work force, paucity of role models, lack of mentorship, inadequate research infrastructure, counseling, and financial support, institutional barriers, and racial discrimination and/or implicit bias that result in isolation or "imposter syndrome" for both URMM surgical trainees and faculty (Fig. 18.1) [13, 29, 30]. In fact, a recent survey of faculty from 26 U.S. medical schools reported that compared to non-URMM faculty, URMM faculty feel like outsiders because of a lack of inclusion, trust, and relationship with their non-minority counterparts [13]. A similar survey of surgical residents confirmed these sentiments, indicating that these feelings begin to evolve during training [14]. In addition, according to Pololi and colleagues, a significant proportion of URMM faculty reported being subjected to racial or ethnic discrimination by a superior, and they also noted a lack of institutional effort to promote equity and diversity. Yet, despite these observations, URMM faculty was more likely to aspire to higher leadership positions than their non-URMM counterparts. However, as noted by the authors, the juxtaposition of high leadership aspirations with the perception of isolation, lack of trust and inclusion predisposes URMM faculty to become disillusioned and to abandon academic medicine completely or miss opportunities for promotion due to discrimination, thus further eroding the pool of future leaders.

Based on the foregoing discussion, URMM surgical leaders face a daunting task. A leader in academic surgery, who happens to be an URMM, has to first establish himself or herself as an academic surgeon. This designation is typically defined by unbiased metrics. In general, those metrics include promotion up the academic ladder, assumption of institutional leadership positions, and national recognition or acknowledgment of the URMM leader's accomplishments by his or her selection for leadership positions by external bodies such as academic surgical societies, boards, national committees, NIH study sections, etc. As noted by Charles Drew, "excellence of performance will transcend artificial barriers created by man" [31]. In addition to establishing his or her credentials as a *bona fide* academic surgeon and earning the respect of his or her peers, the leader in academic surgery who is from an URMM is asked to fill in many roles including: mentor; coach; sponsor; and advocate for URMM surgical trainees and junior faculty by providing them access to growth opportunities (Fig. 18.2). Indeed, the URMM surgical leader has the unique responsibility or duty to serve as a role model for members of his or her underrepresented minority constituency, to help them grow, develop, and to guide them to success. In this context, the URMM mentor or leader

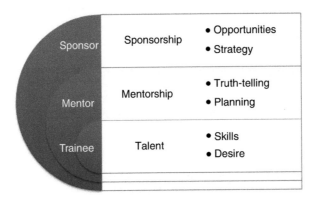

Fig. 18.2 Crucial functions in leadership development. The surgical trainee or future leader is responsible for developing his or her skill set. He or she must have an unwavering commitment to excellence and the desire to succeed. Mentors collaborate with surgical trainees or junior faculty (leaders in development) by coaching, training, supporting, and providing candid advice on choices and performance. Mentors also help develop and monitor the mentee's personal strategic plan. Sponsors recognize talented surgical trainees (emerging future leaders) and provide them access to growth opportunities. Sponsors may also support long strategic maneuvers

must be able to attract, inspire, empower, and ultimately liberate the URMM surgical trainee or mentee to complete the maturation process, while at the same time continuing to advocate for his or her needs, albeit from a distance [12]. Thus, the URMM surgical leader must have a commitment to both mentorship and sponsorship (Fig. 18.3). In essence, URMM surgical leaders have to pay "the minority tax" [32]. The "minority tax" is a complex chain of responsibilities endowed upon minority populations. With this additional burden, URMMs must compete in academia against their colleagues who are not saddled with these requests. Unfortunately, these additional tasks are not always acknowledged as a burden to the URMM. Each additional task for the URMM leads to diminishing satisfaction, lack of promotion, and poor retention. In addition to the added tasks, unconscious bias in workplace, lack of diversity, suboptimal mentorship, institutional racism, professional isolation, and unrelenting clinical duties compound the pressures on the URMM faculty [32]. Ironically, the URMM is then tasked with improving institutional diversity in addition to the standard call of duty. Despite the institutional claims of valuing this diversity, there is often little application of this work as a marker for promotion. And because the URMM may care for the populations that are targets for health disparities more so than the non-URMM, a clinical burden often prevails and thus limiting the URMM from valuable academic or research time. Nevertheless, many URMMs feel the desire to amplify their impact beyond their academic contributions by using their platform to help the local community. They also subscribe to the credo that "EACH ONE REACH ONE" [33]. However, the URMM surgical leader also has a special responsibility to ensure that expanding opportunity for URMM surgical trainees or faculty should never be confused or equated with lowering the standards. There needs to be continued emphasis on

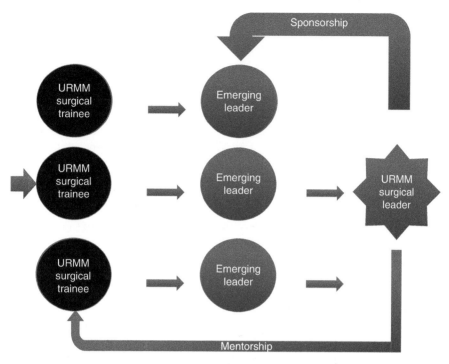

Fig. 18.3 Obligations of an established underrepresented minority leader. URMM surgical leaders have an obligation to develop potential and promote leadership in talented URMM surgical trainees and junior faculty. They should identify promising surgical trainees and junior faculty and provide them access to differing levels of professional challenges and networks at the next level of influence. They also need to find promising talent and mentor them along the path to an emerging leader

the relentless pursuit of excellence and sustained scholarly productivity. URMM mentees have to be prepared to perform "better" than their non-URMM colleagues. URMM surgical leaders must serve as role models for all trainees and colleagues, including students, residents, faculty, deans, presidents and CEOs, to demonstrate that URMM surgeons have made and continue to make significant contributions to the field of surgery. In short, they must have broad appeal to influence the larger sector of society or the surgical community to follow them in expanding opportunities for competent or meritorious URMM surgical trainees and faculty, because, to paraphrase Peter Drucker, there is no leadership without "followership" [34].

To illustrate the foregoing concept, consider how Charles Drew's outstanding research at Columbia University catapulted him to a position of national and international prominence, which put him in position to advocate for a surgical oncology fellowship position for Jack White, the first African-American fellow at Memorial Sloan Kettering Hospital. In turn, Jack White's advocacy later helped LaSalle Leffall obtain a surgical oncology fellowship at Memorial Sloan Kettering Hospital [22, 35]. Dr. Leffall has helped and inspired hundreds, if not thousands, of African-American and other URMM surgeons through his roles as President of the American

Cancer Society, the Society of Surgical Oncology and the American College of Surgeons as well as his 25-year Chairmanship of the Department of Surgery at Howard University [36]. As noted earlier, numerous other African-American surgeons have held leadership positions in mainstream academic societies that invariably helped pave the way for the new generation of contemporary and future URMM surgical leaders. Sam Kountz's brilliance and tenacity paved the way for his election to the Presidency of the Society of University Surgeons. Claude Organ served as Chair of the American Board of Surgery, Chair of the Residency Review Committee, President of the American College of Surgeons, President of the Society of Black Academic Surgeons, and Editor of Archives of Surgery. L.D. Britt is Past President of the American College of Surgeons, the American Surgical Association, the Southern Surgical Society, the American Association for the Surgery of Trauma, and the Society of Black Academic Surgeons. Haile Debas, another prominent URMM academic surgical leader, served as Dean of the University of California at San Francisco, President of the American Surgical Association, and President of the Society of Black Academic Surgeons. Steven Stain is former Chair of the American Board of Surgery and past president of the Society of Black Academic Surgeons. Henri R. Ford served as President of the Association for Academic Surgery, the Surgical Infection Society, and the Society of Black Academic Surgeons. Lastly, Fiemu Nwarieku is a past president of the Association for Academic Surgery. The significant increase in the number of African-American chairs of departments of surgery and deans of U.S. medical schools in recent years is arguably directly related to the contributions made by previous URMM surgical leaders who were the trailblazers in academic surgery.

The historical achievements of past surgical heroes impart important lessons for leaders confronting present struggles. Their memory is perpetuated in quotes, named lectures, named services, streets, buildings, institutions, etcetera. They privately and publicly worked to move systems in order to construct foundations for new opportunities. They include the late legacies who posthumously educate and mentor the academic surgeons who follow. Also, not forgotten are our current giants in leadership who are shaping the present. They engage in active, meaningful community service as an essential component in their portfolio. They exercise their influence to address, at a policy level, the problems or challenges that limit the pipeline of URMM students achieving the necessary proficiency in reading, math and science to enable them to ultimately be competitive for medical school. They combat racial and ethnic prejudice as well as other barriers that hinder upward social mobility, promote and champion diversity, and lobby for improved access to quality health care for underserved communities while serving as visible role models and as a source of inspiration for their underrepresented minority constituencies. Such grassroots advocacy is a *sine qua non* in order to ultimately reduce or eliminate health disparities. Hence, the responsibilities of URMM surgical leaders are profound.

In summary, the pathway to becoming a leader in academic surgery is challenging in general given the stressors of health care economics, clinical workload and burnout. For URMMs the addition of other social barriers such as discrimination, lack of mentorship, and financial burdens pose additional challenges to reaching the highest leadership positions in academic surgery. Contemporary URMM surgical leaders must also recognize that whatever stature they have achieved in American surgery is the result of the legacy of excellence and advocacy of past URMM trailblazers such as Drs. Drew, Kountz, Leffall, and Organ. Yet these individuals were invariably aided along their journey by non-URMM mentors and sponsors who recognized their brilliance and gave them an opportunity to shine. Although current URMM surgical leaders should accept to pay the "color tax" of role modeling, mentoring, sponsoring or enhancing opportunities for other URMM surgical trainees and faculty, their leadership should recognize this additional burden and make sure they do their part to support the success of these individuals and the community they are serving. Today, we are reminded that our predecessors faced far greater obstacles in climbing to success in spite of a paucity of role models, mentors and sponsors. They in some ways with far less resources and access to social media had to pay a much greater and more stressful tax in order for us to enjoy the privilege of reaching the highest echelon of American surgery. Indeed, these obstacles are apparent as the building blocks of adversity that define and, invariably, refine the minority leader in academic surgery.

Acknowledgment The authors wish to thank the following outstanding leaders in academic surgery, who happen to be from an underrepresented minority in medicine, for their continuing support, mentoring, and insightful contributions to this chapter: L.D. Britt, Andre Campbell, Edward Cornwell, Steven Stain, Patricia Turner, and Selwyn Vickers.

References

1. IOM. How far have we come in reducing health disparities?: Progress since 2000: workshop summary. Washington, DC: The National Academies Press; 2012.
2. U.S. Department of Health and Human Services, Agency for Healthcare Research and Quality. National healthcare disparities report. Rockville, MD: AHRQ; 2014.
3. AAMC. Diversity in medical education: facts & figures 2012. Association of American Medical Colleges, Diversity Policy and Programs. Washington, DC: AAMC; 2012. p. 20.
4. Butler PD, Longaker MT, Britt LD. Addressing the paucity of underrepresented minorities in academic surgery: can the "Rooney Rule" be applied to academic surgery? Am J Surg. 2010;199:255–62.
5. Jenkins RR. Diversity and inclusion: strategies to improve pediatrics and pediatric health care delivery. Pediatrics. 2014;133:327–30.
6. United States Census Bureau. State & county QuickFacts. Suitland, MD: United States Census Bureau; 2014.
7. AAMC. Total enrollment by U.S. Medical School and race and ethnicity, 2013. Washington, DC: Association of American Medical Colleges; 2014.
8. AAMC. Distribution of U.S. medical school faculty by sex, race/hispanic origin, tenure status, and department. Washington, DC: Association of American Medical Colleges; 2014.
9. AAMC. Number of active residents, by type of medical school, GME specialty, and sex, 2016–2017. Washington, DC: Association of American Medical Colleges; 2017.
10. United States Census Bureau. Annual resident population estimates of the United States by race and Hispanic or Latino origin: April 1, 2000 to July 1, 2002. Suitland, MD: United States Census Bureau; 2002.

11. United States Census Bureau. Annual estimates of the resident population by sex, race, and Hispanic origin for the United States: April 1, 2010 to July 1, 2011. Suitland, MD: United States Census Bureau; 2011.
12. Ford HR. Mentoring, diversity, and academic surgery. J Surg Res. 2004;118:1–8.
13. Pololi LH, Evans AT, Gibbs BK, Krupat E, Brennan RT, et al. The experience of minority faculty who are underrepresented in medicine, at 26 representative U.S. medical schools. Acad Med. 2013;88:1308–14.
14. Wong RL, Sullivan MC, Yeo HL, Roman SA, Bell RH, et al. Race and surgical residency: results from a national survey of 4339 US general surgery residents. Ann Surg. 2013;257:782–7.
15. Williams DH. Stab wound of the heart and pericardium - suture of the pericardium - recovery - patient alive three years afterward. Am Period Med Rec. 1897;51:437.
16. Cobb WM. Daniel Hale Williams-Pioneer and Innovator. J Natl Med Assoc. 1944;36:158–9.
17. Organ CH Jr. A century of black surgeons: the U.S.A. experience. Norman, OK: Transcript Press; 1987.
18. Cornwell EE. Dr. Asa Yancey and the realization of his mentor's dream. Bull Am Coll Surg. 2016;101:53–4.
19. Yancey AG, Cromartie JE, Ford JR, Nichols RR, Saville AF. A modification of the Swenson technique for congenital megacolon. J Natl Med Assoc. 1952;44:356–63.
20. Organ CH. The black surgeon in the twentieth century: a tribute to Samuel L. Kountz, MD. J Natl Med Assoc. 1978;70:683–4.
21. Brown DL. Changing the face of medicine. Bethesda, MD: US National Library of Medicine.
22. Schneidman DS. Breaking down barriers for minorities and cancer patients: a profile of LaSalle D. Leffall, Jr. Bull Am Coll Surg. 2011;96:18–24.
23. Organ CH Jr. Opening doors: contemporary African American Academic Surgeons. Bethesda, MD: U.S. National Library of Medicine; 2006.
24. Organ CH Jr. A century of back surgeons: the U.S.A experience. Norman, OK: Transcript Press; 1987.
25. Simpson E. Respected Suffolk surgeon takes prestigious position. The Virgininan-Pilot. Norfolk, VA: Landmark Media Enterprises L.L.C.; 2010. http://hamptonroads.com/2010/2009/respected-suffolk-surgeon-takes-prestigious-position.
26. New Frontiers in Academic Surgery. Opening doors: contemporary African American Academic Surgeons. Bethesda, MD: U.S. National Library of Medicine; 2006.
27. Alvord LA. Changing the face of medicine. Bethesda, MD: National Library of Medicine.
28. Quiñones-Hinojosa A. Illegal farm worker becomes brain surgeon. Washington, DC: National Public Radio; 2011.
29. Pololi L, Cooper LA, Carr P. Race, disadvantage and faculty experiences in academic medicine. J Gen Intern Med. 2010;25:1363–9.
30. Chapman EN, Kaatz A, Carnes M. Physicians and implicit bias: how doctors may unwittingly perpetuate health care disparities. J Gen Intern Med. 2013;28:1504–10.
31. Leffall LD. Seven surgical exemplars and the College--lest we forget. Am J Surg. 1998;176:361–5.
32. Gonzalez P, Stoll B. The color of medicine: strategies for increasing diversity in the U.S. physician workforce. Boston, MA: Community Catalyst; 2002.
33. Waymer D. Each one, reach one: an autobiographic account of a Black PR professor's mentor-mentee relationships with Black graduate students. Pub Relat Inq. 2012;1:398–414.
34. Kruse K. What is leadership? Jersey City, NJ: ForbesForbes.com LLC; 2013. http://www.forbes.com/sites/kevinkruse/2013/2004/2009/what-is-leadership/.
35. Cornwell EE, III. Personal correspondence. 29 September 2014.
36. Copeland EM. LaSalle D. Leffall, Jr., MD, FACS: the first Heritage Award winner, Society of Surgical Oncology. Ann Surg Oncol. 2001;8:477–9.

Index

© Springer Nature Switzerland AG 2019
M. R. Kibbe, H. Chen (eds.), *Leadership in Surgery*, Success in Academic
Surgery, https://doi.org/10.1007/978-3-030-19854-1